THE WELLNESS METHOD

ONE YEAR FROM NOW, YOU WILL BE HAPPY YOU STARTED TODAY!

DR. BRADLEY KOBSAR, DC, DACBN AND
JUDY PEARSON KOBSAR, CHHC, CWP

DEDICATION

In writing this dedication we know without a doubt that the Creator brought the two of us together with the divine purpose of blazing a trail so that others can be well. We are humbled by this calling on our hearts and intend to honor our Creator through the health that will be delivered to the many.

To our precious daughters who teach us every day what it means to purposefully guide souls through this life. Who inspire us to reach higher, go further and love deeper.

To our parents, our mentors, and our spiritual leaders who have guided us, coached us, and lead us to become the highest versions of our selves to help us fulfill our calling.

To our Wellness Method Team and our many Wellness Partners who's commitment to health inspires us to grow and serve with excellence.

TABLE OF CONTENTS

The Wellness Method

One Year from Now, You Will Be Happy You Started Today!

*"In 365 days, you will replace 98% of your cells - you
literally recreate your body every year. Your choices TODAY
will determine the health of your cells tomorrow."*

~ Dr. Brad Kobsar

Congratulations on taking your first step toward recreating your health, your youth and your life. If you are reading this book, we want to personally commend you on moving forward and taking responsibility for your most valuable asset: your health and well-being.

By reading this book, you have the opportunity to not only make a difference in your life, but to make a difference in the lives of those you love, and who love and depend on you. Prepare for a life-changing experience that will empower you to take charge of your health and live the abundant life you were destined to live!

Dr. Bradley Kobsar's Story:

Stage 4 Cancer, End Stage Diabetes and Liver failure. This is what I was facing in 1995 when I was hired to create and direct the first Wellness Program in the Santa Clara County Hospital System. I had just received a 5-year grant in collaboration with the County Hospital's chronic disease clinic. The Chronic Disease Clinic was a hard place to work. There were a lot of people suffering with nausea, vomiting, inability to sleep or eat; and eventually for too many, loss of life. The grant award came from the federal government and the state of California to implement my Wellness program and the incredible visionary leadership at the County Health and Hospital system to recognize the need for this. We hit the ground running and in no time, I had a 12-week waiting list because the doctors saw their patients who were in my program turning their health and their lives around; so I was flooded with referrals.

I was even hired by pharmaceutical companies to do wellness presentations all over Northern California, which I was happy to do. This was my passion: to educate people about how to take care of their health through natural methods rather than needing to rely on medications, doctors, and health insurance. But I was a little puzzled because I didn't prescribe medications ... so why would Merck, Dupont, Bristol Meyers and other big pharmaceutical companies want to hire me? Well, it turned out that I was good for their business. You see, before going through my Wellness Program, the patients were so sick from the toxic side effects of the drugs that they just refused to take them altogether. The medications made them sicker than the actual disease they were suffering from, so they just stopped. After going through my wellness program, they felt so much better that you'll never guess what happened next! They were put back on their medications! That's right, I had gotten the patients healthier and then they were better able to tolerate the side effects of the medications, so they were put back on all their drugs.

Well, as you can imagine the wellness doctor inside me was not ecstatic to discover this. I tried to focus on the positive benefits that the patients and I had achieved together, but after this same pattern repeated over the course of 5 years, I could no longer stand by and watch patients have their liver shut down or be forced onto dialysis from toxic kidney failure and then pass away a few weeks later. My hands were tied, and as heartbreaking as it was, I turned down more grant funding and moved on into private practice. There is a happy ending here- many of my patients followed me and I was able to care for them on my terms, and it changed their lives. I left to go into private practice because didn't want any more interference from the health care system, and 20 years later I am gratified to say that many lives have been changed, and in some cases it meant the difference between life and death for those patients. I stopped calling them 'patients' and began calling them Wellness Partners, because we are true partners in their health care and I can spend as much time as needed, and order all necessary tests. This is the approach that I use today to help scores of people just like you change your life.

Many years later I met Judy Pearson Kobsar. She came to me as an injured dancer with the impending doom of having to retire far too soon from the art she loved. After being a patient, then business partner, then friend and eventually my wife, we saw that together we could do great things to help people restore their health. There are many reasons why writing this book was such a high priority for us. The biggest reason is that it is so hard to get helpful education in our healthcare system because no one has time to talk to patients in the average 7-10 minute appointment. We have always loved working directly with people to restore their health, and dreamed about writing a book that would help others who are struggling with their health.

I always felt that as a full time working doctor, it would be incredibly difficult to find the time to write a book. With a full-time practice, 2 kids, a wife and my sleep demands, I thought becoming an author would be impossible. How could I achieve that dream? The best chance of writing a book would be by waking up two hours prior to my usual rising time, and write. So here I am in the dark of the early morning . . . doing the impossible: waking up a couple hours before work or finding the energy and focus at the end of a long work day to come home, spend time with my girls, and then find the creativity to sit down and start writing! I am driven to help people gain wellness, and know that there is valuable information inside of me that just has to get out to the world.

Warm regards,

DR. BRADLEY KOBSAR DC, DACBN
Certified Functional Medicine Practitioner
Board Certified in Clinical Nutrition
Board Certified Chiropractor
Founder, The Wellness Method

Judy's Story

Literally crawling in to a Chiropractor's clinic from a back injury was my first introduction to Holistic and Wellness care. I grew up the daughter of a Medical Technologist, so any time there was a cold, flu, ailment of any kind we were medicated, or we went to the medical clinic. I am grateful for the care I received because of my mother's degree and position, but I did not know at the time that there was any other way to heal the body. I abruptly woke up to Holistic and Wellness care the day I hobbled in to have my first Chiropractic Exam. What? No medications? You aren't prescribing meds? I'm doing what? Coming in here to get bodywork done? Lifting weights?? Eating differently? Learning about my pain and injury? Huh? This was how I met Dr. Bradley Kobsar back in 2005.

If you can imagine, it was like learning a whole new language for me. I thought I was a stud . . . I mean I had received athletic awards all through my life, I was currently an Artistic Director of a major dance company and less than 2 months away from putting my show up on stage. Just give me Advil and I'll be on my way! Trouble was, I couldn't even walk, let alone dance, and I feared I had directed and danced my last show ever—it was devastating. I had never experienced an injury like this in my life, and I didn't understand it. As athletic as I was, I knew nothing about the human body. So, though reserved, I began to embrace this new method of healing, and to my surprise not only did I heal, but I became a stronger dancer and athlete than I was in my 20's and 30's . . . and I was 40 at the time of my injury! I fell in love with this approach and dove into learning as much as I could. Little did I know, many years later we would be married, running our Wellness Method clinic, and helping thousands of people all across the country restore their health.

Once I understood Dr. Kobsar's approach- that the body has the ability to heal given the right support- and was completely restored through it, I became hungry for more knowledge and education. I got certified as a personal trainer and Pilates instructor, I went to nutrition school to become a certified nutritionist and holistic health coach, I opened my own personal training business, health coaching practice, and then years later went into business with Dr. Kobsar, running our wellness center in San Jose, California. I continued to dance, produce and choreograph for many years after my injury, and currently today at 53 years old, though no longer on stage, I am healthier now than I was prior to my injury. Life throws us curves, but there are always reasons and meaning in the curves if we can be open to seeing them. That injury, though devastating, changed the trajectory of my life and brought me here, to writing this book that will reach countless seekers of health!

Dr. Kobsar and I have evolved our wellness practice and philosophies over many years to what we have always dreamed would be a program that is accessible to anyone, anywhere in the world at any age, who wishes to restore and recreate their health and live the life they desire. It is called The Wellness Method, and we want to share it with you.

Warm Regards,

JUDY PEARSON KOBSAR, CHHC, CWP
Certified Nutritionist
Longevity Wellness Specialist

THE WELLNESS METHOD

The Wellness Method is based on our 8 Principles of Wellness. If these foundational principles are in your life on a regular basis, you can't help but turn your health around and recreate your life. Once you begin restoring your health, your entire life begins to change for the better. This is our simple, yet scientifically proven approach that has breathed life into so many others, and you could be next! The 8 Principles are:

Regimen
Educational Curriculum
Coaching
Reducing Inflammation
Endocrine System
Alignment of Your Structure
Total Nutrition
Exercise

It's no accident that our Principles spell **"RECREATE"**. We call our principles **"RECREATE 365"** to honor the body's ability to renew itself in 365 days. Our scientifically proven system follows a step by step process to improve the function of your body as a whole and

RECREATE your health. Your body is forever renewing itself and regenerating cells; in fact, one year from now you are going to replace 98% of the cells in your body. Every cell in your body turns over while at the same time your body is destroying old cells. The only exception is your brain and nerve cells– they turn over at a much slower rate so they don't really cause any significant difference. So, knowing that every day a billion of your cells die, but every day a billion new cells are produced, there is a lot of power in that because YOU get to determine the health of those new cells based on the choices you make about the way you live. If you continue to live recklessly, not taking care of yourself, the new cells will not be vital cells and you'll be more prone to disease. But if you start now, restoring your health-your body will respond, and those cells will be regenerating in the healthiest way possible!

Look at the Wisdom of the Body - It is Truly Powerful!

In 6 days you will have a new stomach lining.
In 3 months you will have a new skeleton.
In 6 months you will have a new liver.
In 1 year you will have a new you.

What Do You Want The New Version Of You To Be?

Will you be healthier, or in continued decline? Some skeptics might think that if we are getting new cells every day, then they are exactly that-'new' . . . so they will be the same or even better. We've also heard people say, "Well if I'm getting new cells, then they are renewing in the same condition as the old ones- so, I'm just going to stay the same and not get any worse." That sounds fine in theory, but the truth of the matter is you are aging and unfortunately that does not work in your favor unless you are actively doing something to ensure that your health is improving. If your car needs an oil change or the brakes replaced, and you do nothing, after one year is it going to be better or worse? Worse of course. So if you do nothing, in one year your joints will have more wear and tear and your brain and heart will have the effects of another year of stress. Will it be healthy stress causing you to thrive or unhealthy stress causing inflammation and degeneration? You recreate yourself every day with the choices you make of how you want to live.

Why are the RECREATE Principles Crucial?

Long-term predictions for chronic diseases keep rising due to physical, emotional, and mental stress from diet, emotions, environment, drugs, injuries, accidents, lack of sleep, lack of exercise, and our generally unhealthy overly stressed lifestyles. Our 8 Principles work to keep you from being a high-risk candidate for disease. The rule is simple: Prevent disease now so there's nothing to "treat" later. Diabetes, cardiovascular damage, thyroid disease, cancer, autoimmune conditions, and even back problems can take months and years to form into a health compromising issue. Chronic disease is typically slow to develop, but the good news is you have time to resolve your issues by making some simple changes. So, if you already happen to be riding the risk-rollercoaster of disease (typical for people over 30), you can start reversing the acquired stress damage by enabling your body to heal itself. This is a very different approach than the 'conventional' approach to suppressing signs of disease or masking symptoms with medications.

The Wellness Method focuses on resolving the *underlying causes of health issues* rather than treating symptoms. Our approach emphasizes treatment of the *person*, NOT the disease. The Wellness Method is a partnership between doctor and patient. The Wellness Method is a *complement* to conventional medicine where the two systems of health can work together wherever possible. We recognize that one approach cannot serve everyone's needs all of the time, therefore we want to share with you each of our 8 Principles in detail, so that you can implement them in your life and witness the changes for yourself.

"Without education, you can't bring wellness to those that are seeking it. And you can't bring wellness to those who are not ready . . . regardless of how much they are in need."

~ Dr. Brad Kobsar, DC, DACBN

We come in to contact with two types of people in our industry:

1. The person who desperately needs help, is on several medications, living a compromised life but is not emotionally ready to make a change.
2. The person who is living the same compromised life but is desperate for change! They have tried many different things and are frustrated with the lack of results and are looking for help.

Both types of people need help, and both need education, but type #1 requires a mental shift or maybe a crisis before they will seek help and even that does not always move them to action. Type #2 typically comes to us very frustrated and losing hope but are ready to change!

Have you ever tried to improve your health through diet or exercise or by taking hormone replacement therapy or some other method? Have you gotten some positive results only to see your efforts stall, become stagnant, or maybe even turn in the wrong direction? Did you wonder why this happened? Why, despite your best efforts, you didn't achieve your goals? We know so many have experienced this frustrating cycle—for this reason, education is always the first step to help them understand WHY there was failure, that most of the time it isn't their fault, and really all they need is a plan, structure and an element of support.

As shared earlier, each letter of RECREATE represents a step in our method. Each step or principle can fill a book on its own but our intent here is to give you a good solid foundation of our approach so that you can start making measurable changes in your life immediately and see results you never thought possible! The system must be followed together with all foundations intact however— you do not want to leave any of the principles out.

Simply put, if you do not address these 8 Principles together, your efforts will most likely fail. A wise man once said, "If you fail to prepare, you are preparing to fail." If you only address a portion of our 8 Principles of health, you will get a 'portion' of the results. Our intent is to give you a comprehensive approach to putting all of the pieces of our method together. Let's take a look at the importance of each component and its role in optimized health with a broad overview of each Principle. Then we will take a deep dive into each principle with dedicated chapters.

OVERVIEW OF THE PRINCIPLES OF THE WELLNESS METHOD: RECREATE 365

REGIMEN

94% of people fail because there is no system or structure in place and most plans are not comprehensive. In the past 20 years, I have seen Nutritionists doing personal training and Personal Trainers doing nutrition, however neither are trained or licensed to interpret Labs, or to manage Injuries, Hormones and Detox programs. I've seen Doctor's offices manage Hormones, Detox programs and *sometimes* nutrition but they don't oversee and evaluate exercise programs or treat injuries other than with anti-inflammation medications. Missing just one of the 8 RECREATE Principles can stop you in your tracks. Missing two of the Principles is certain failure. It breaks our hearts when we see people working hard and following instructions, but they are missing too many pieces and they've wasted a lot of time and in many cases a lot of money on a plan that just wasn't comprehensive and complete. Then they begin to lose hope and become frustrated.

You could have a hormone imbalance that sabotages your weight loss even when you are doing everything right! But your personal trainer or your nutritionist can't diagnose that, and you'll be running into a brick wall over and over until you get labs done and a correct diagnosis. Insulin resistance from blood sugar instability, low Testosterone, a stomach that can't absorb nutrients, or an injury from exercise . . . all of these are often overlooked without a comprehensive health and wellness strategy and often results in frustration and quitting. And who do you blame? Usually yourself. But it's not your fault. You needed a comprehensive and structured program with all principals addressed so you can have complete success in all areas of your health. When you read the chapter on Regimen, you will understand the value of a proven system, and why it will ensure your success.

EDUCATION

If you are going to learn anything new, there will always be an order to your learning. We call this a Curriculum. If you are going to learn to restore your health through the Wellness Method 8 RECREATE Method Principles, then you need to be educated. Just like if you were to learn to fly a plane . . . you must learn it, practice it, have a guide and mentor, study it, own it and embed it in your life. Then you will have it forever, and with our method you will be able to pass it on to your family and your loved ones. We have talked to so many that have failed because they tried to restore their health without truly learning about the processes of their own body, without learning about their conditions and the remedies, without learning what is right for their individual nutritional needs and the detailed aspects of their path to health. It's hard to watch, because we know that even if they make some progress, they eventually regress and often quit trying. What is critical to understand about the Education Principle is that you must be convicted in your desire to invest in yourself.

We invest years, time and our money into college, trade schools, job advancement courses and equipment to 'make a living'. But what we see is that most people are "Living to Work" instead of "Working to Live". Working to Live means that THE QUALITY OF YOUR LIFE is more important than anything. And your income/work-life should support a high quality of health-related living. But what we most often see is that people work so hard just to pay the bills or to accumulate 'things' while completely sacrificing their health and quality of life. We witness people missing out on time with their children or grandchildren only to age with chronic disease and disabilities because they did not invest in themselves along the way. It is time to shift your thinking about investing in yourself and understand that this is not the time or place to 'bargain hunt and find a good deal.' Infact this is the time to put forth great effort, resources and focus into your health. We will get into deeper detail about the Educational Principle and investing in yourself in a later chapter. In addition, education about our current health care system is an important part of the Education Principle. You must understand where you've been to clearly see where you must go, to get the results you are so desperately searching for.

COACHING

You can have all the tools, systems, gadgets, downloads, software and information, but if your mindset is not aligned with restoring your health and making changes that will RECREATE your life, then none of those things matter and you will sabotage yourself before you even get out of the gate. Mindset is everything. First, we must address where your mindset is currently, and then we have to 'shift' your mindset to a winning state that will support your journey to Recreate your health. When you learn something new you need a guide. When you learn to fly a plane, you study the Law of Lift and read about the mechanics of the plane, you take classes, you have an instructor, watch videos and you would practice in a simulator. And then, eventually you're ready to get in the plane and take it up in the air. But who would you want with you in the cockpit when you are learning to fly? Yes! Your instructor. You need a mentor to guide you. Learning to restore your health is the same.

It's human nature to do things subconsciously to sabotage and override the conscious mind because it has been a habit. This is why you may find yourself frustrated with not having any 'willpower' to change the things you know are not good for you, that keep you up at night because of unwanted thoughts you can't get out of your mind. Willpower really is an overused word that doesn't hold much weight when it comes to restoring your health. You must change your habits; and to do this, you must first change your mindset. Because even though what you are doing at that moment is painful to you, and you desire change- it is not as painful as changing that habit. Everyone needs a coach to help make changes - we have coaches and mentors that support us in our lives. Infact, one of our trusted mentors introduced us to the concept of focusing on 'mind-shift' rather than 'mind-set'. In the Coaching Chapter, you will learn exercises to begin shifting your mindset that support healthy changes in your life.

REDUCE INFLAMMATION

Every day, we breathe in chemicals in the air, allergens and smog. We drink water that is often full of chemicals meant to "clean" it that are hormone disruptors which affect our body functions. We eat and drink processed products that affect our digestion and our natural detoxification processes and capacities. This is simply a part of life in our modern, industrialized society but it is causing inflammation in our body.

Your body has natural detoxification processes that are working 24/7. The liver is your main detoxification organ, but you also naturally detoxify through your kidneys, bowels, sweat glands and respiratory system. These chemical stressors you endure, and your daily choices often hinder and impede the function of your detoxification systems which adversely affects your bodily functions. A proper and complete detoxification system does not simply consist of a bowel cleanse or juicing as many people believe. All of the detoxification system pathways must be addressed in a proper method to ensure optimal function, lower inflammation and improve overall health. Then they must be maintained and nurtured to provide insurance that bodily functions work at an optimal level. We will teach you all about how and why toxins affect the systems of your body and what to do to reduce them in your life on a regular basis.

ENDOCRINE SYSTEM (Hormones)

Hormones are the chemical messengers that communicate within your body. There are hundreds of different hormones that work daily to make your body a well-oiled machine as they regulate everything in your body: sex properties and function, energy production, metabolism, lean muscle promotion, mood, sleep, body composition and more. Small abnormalities or imbalances will throw off regulatory balance and cause poor communication which inevitably leads to poor health. The imbalance or decline can occur rapidly or slowly over years and will affect many other systems along the way. Poor diet, hygiene, stress (both external and internal), toxicity, lack of exercise, structural issues, pain and everyday life affect your hormone balance both positively and negatively.

If hormones are not properly evaluated and brought into balance, optimal health is not obtainable. Hormone balance is essential for proper organ/gland function, which means it is essential for proper metabolism, weight maintenance, energy production, sleep, digestion, mood and so much more. The hormones of the brain are called neurotransmitters. You may have heard about serotonin, dopamine, GABA, acetylcholine. These chemicals allow your brain to run efficiently.

ALIGNMENT of Your Structure

Structure consists of bones, joints, ligaments, muscles and your nervous system. As you move thru daily life activities, the integration of all these structural parts work to provide you the ability to be mobile. When there is a malfunction or misalignment in any one of your structures, the other structural parts must compensate for this. This creates a kinetic chain of events that reprogram and rewire throughout your entire structure until it is reset for normal, healthy function. When this fails to occur, problems gradually creep up and if allowed to continue create chronic problems in your joints, muscles and nerves. If nerve impulses are too low or too high, it causes pain, numbness, tingling, spasm, weakness, etc. all of which start a debilitating path to structural degeneration.

Structural care is a largely overlooked aspect of health. Over time muscle weaknesses, postural imbalances, injuries, neglect and inactivity lead to compromised function and degenerative changes. Your body is made to move. Structural degeneration (arthritis, joint pain, muscle pain etc.) is not a problem of age as we are often told, it is an issue of proper function. Malfunction of the nervous system and structural integrity lowers our potential for health and affect all aspects of our biological functions adversely.

TOTAL NUTRITION

Have you ever gone on a diet plan and lost weight, only to have a rebound weight gain of more weight than you lost? Many of the fad diets or diet programs where they send you your food are very often filled with processed and preserved foods. While these plans may provide short term weight loss, they can take a toll on your overall health and hormones functions. Why? Because they don't provide the right nutrition for your body to grow, build, repair, and function. Fad diets and counting calories usually ends with hormone imbalance, toxification and poor health.

You will learn that as an individual, you have your own specific needs that are unique to you, your body, your health concerns and your health goals. We all need nutrients but we also must understand what foods work for us and what foods work against us as individuals. This chapter will give you a deep understanding into why diets and counting calories don't work and how you can begin to determine what proper nutrition is for you specifically.

EXERCISE

Our body was meant to move. It is meant to be in motion. That is why it is constructed the way it is constructed. We have joints and bones, and muscles that are meant to be used. We stand erect because we are meant to carry loads and use our frame and structure provided to get things done. When we neglect our body and don't exercise it, we begin to break down, lose muscle tone, become weak and flaccid and we suffer. The good news is that a good exercise program doesn't have to involve the same training as a professional athlete. You can transform your body, gain lean muscle, and burn unwanted fat in as little as a few sessions per week, if you are using the right methods and program. Proper coaching and information is necessary for us all to achieve our goals. We provide that information and education here in this book. When you understand that exercise and weight bearing activities are essential to obtaining optimal health, you will have the tools to transform your body, to look your best and to become healthier.

Why Do You Need The Wellness Method's 8 Principles of RECREATE 365?

Our society is experiencing a sharp increase in the number of people who suffer from chronic diseases, such as diabetes, heart disease, cancer and autoimmune disease. 'Chronic disease' is the term the medical system gave to conditions that go unresolved and continue on and on without any resolution. Hypothyroidism, chronic fatigue, fibromyalgia, irritable bowels, are more of these chronic conditions that our conventional medical system does not have a 'cure' for. We purposefully did not capitalize the titles of these conditions because we want you to understand they do not deserve a permanent place in our dictionaries, nor in our lives. And it's critical for you to understand that 50 years ago none of these conditions existed. Let that sink in a moment. 50 Years ago none of these conditions existed so it's clear we have created these conditions because of the way we live along with the insurance-based healthcare system's inability to resolve root causes of these conditions. Medications do not resolve the root cause of illness, medication treat symptoms. This is a key point for you to understand in order to adopt the mindset necessary to restore your health.

Our system of healthcare is designed to address acute care, which is the diagnosis and treatment of trauma, or disease through urgent care such as appendicitis or a fractured bone. Doctors apply treatments like drugs or surgery to treat the immediate problem which works fine for those situations but unfortunately, the acute-care approach lacks the methods and tools for preventing and treating complex, chronic disease and everyday health issues. It does not take into account the unique biology and genetic makeup of each individual or factors such as environmental exposure to toxins. The current systems does not account for the factors of today's lifestyle that influence the rise in common health issues like high blood pressure and chronic disease. In other words, our current healthcare is a 'one-size-fits-all' approach to treat disease, instead of treating you.

The Wellness Method is an evolution in the practice of healthcare by shifting the current 'disease-centered' focus of healthcare to a 'patient-centered' approach. We designed this method to address the whole person, not just symptoms. We've been practicing this way for over 20 years and by spending far more than the average 15-minute appointment time, we get a deeper understanding of you and your health concerns. We run lab tests that tell us the underlying cause of your problem (not just what medication to take) and we then create a plan to restore health not just treat symptoms. We focus on the interactions of your genetics along with your environment and lifestyle factors which influence long-term health and chronic disease. We then work together as Wellness Partners (not patients) on your health care. In this way, each of the 8 RECREATE 365 Principles support the unique expression of health and vitality for each individual. YOU are an individual, and your healthcare should reflect what is unique and different about you.

There's a huge gap between current research and our conventional healthcare approach. This gap is enormous—as much as 50 years—particularly in the area of chronic disease. Medical schools are not adequately training doctors to assess the underlying causes of health issues. Medical schools do not teach strategies in the areas of nutrition, diet, and exercise to treat, and prevent illness. By learning The Wellness Method, YOU will learn the steps to resolving many of your health problems. We have helped thousands of our Wellness Partners literally rewrite the story of their lives with this method, now it's your turn! So let's dive into each Principle along with some action steps that you can begin taking action immediately to recreate, restore and reclaim your health!

REGIMEN

Regimen
Educational Curriculum
Coaching
Reducing Inflammation
Endocrine System
Alignment of Your Structure
Total Nutrition
Exercise

A well put together Regimen should provide a system or a step by step approach with a path to follow so it is simple to re-create a more healthy and vital you. This is our chief aim with this book—for you to come away with a Personalized Health Regimen for yourself. We created The Wellness Method to address the systems of your body by implementing a system that addresses inflammation control, diet and nutrition, muscle and joint health, exercise physiology, detoxification, hormone balancing and genetic risk management. With this **R**egimen, you will have a complete and comprehensive path to the health you desire.

There are many practitioners we've observed who are addressing just a few pieces of total health, not the entire system of the body. We see doctors prescribe only drugs and surgery, we watch nutritionists cover only diet, calories in/out and maybe detoxification, we've witnessed fitness instructors focus on exercise and maybe some basic nutrition, and we know chiropractors and physical therapists that help your bone and joint health, but that is it. We understand that the reason they are only able to focus on these few elements of care is because that is their acquired expertise. The problem in these approaches is that they are not addressing the total YOU. If your only tool is a hammer, everything looks like a nail and there's only one tool to get that nail pounded in. But what's not being addressed is all the issues that surround the nail. So in your body, problems persist because the work is being done in just specific compartments of your health, instead of your total health. If you are one of the rare lucky ones to have a simple cause with a simple solution, that's great. If diet and exercise get you results, awesome! If you sprain your wrist or change your posture that's a simple problem with a simple fix. Sadly, for most people, they have complex problems. You might be one of these people, so you might continue to suffer for years, or maybe you've already been suffering for years. There is more going on than what meets the eye and deeper investigation is required.

Why Treating Symptoms is a Recipe for Disaster

Having a regimen, a plan, a path to restoring your health is the only way to truly recreate your health and your life. If you still believe your doctor is improving your health conditions because he or she has prescribed medication, we'd like to suggest you open your mind to understanding what true healing is. Doctors are very well-trained to treat symptoms, but NOT to address the causes of illness. We are intently focused and interested in ALL of your symptoms, because they are the clues to seeing your deeper imbalances. Once we find those deeper imbalances and correct them together, healing begins to occur naturally, and the symptoms resolve along with underlying cause of the problem.

This is the key to our Wellness Method which is based in Functional Medicine. This approach could save your life because it looks at all parts of your body- all of your systems, not just one organ system. Functional Medicine has also been called Systems Medicine because we discover the dysfunction of ALL the <u>systems</u> to restore your body's natural ability to heal. Functional Medicine improves the function of your body as a whole. Unfortunately, conventional medicine doesn't work that way. If a depressed patient also has an infection, for example, he is sent to an internist. If the same patient has a stomach problem, he is sent to a gastroenterologist. Sleep issue? See a sleep specialist. And from each doctor, he gets the 'right' approach for each individual problem, with no one looking at how all these symptoms, including the depression, are connected and how addressing the underlying cause can help everything. So the patient ends up being treated with the 'right' medications for the specific symptoms - but is still sick!

Disease Centered Healthcare

Our health care in the US costs us twice as much as any other country in the world, so . . . ***Why aren't we the healthiest country in the world?!*** This is a question that we all should be asking ourselves every day and not resting until we resolve this imbalance- but sadly, our country has become numb to the large and disturbing disparity between what health care costs us, and how sick our country is. We've 'accepted' it and with that, we've accepted a compromised life riddled with chronic disease, disabilities, illness, depression and a myriad of new diagnosis that come up each year.

"What we accept to be true will define our path in life. Accept nothing but the very best for your health and your path will be filled with restoration, opportunity for change, and vitality!"

~ Judy Pearson Kobsar

A Note From Dr. Kobsar

When you are given a medical 'diagnosis', it doesn't necessarily mean you now know what's wrong with you. We know that might be hard for you to believe, and we didn't believe it either . . . but it is true. As a doctor, I was trained to think that people with the same diagnosis were the same and should be treated the same. That means I was trained to believe that one person's neuropathy was the same as someone else's neuropathy, and that obesity was the same for everyone. There is something so foundationally wrong with this approach, and over the past 75 years, we have seen the negative repercussions of it on our people, communities and dear family members. When doctors practice with this thought process, we end up treating the disease — not the CAUSE. The truth is, everyone is different, even people with the same disease diagnosis, therefore we must look to the ROOT CAUSE of the disease and the individual at a deeper level in order to truly RESOLVE their health issue.

The Corporate Playbook To Healthcare

The conventional approach to health care is causing our global obesity, diabetes and heart disease epidemics to rise every year. One in two Americans has pre-diabetes or diabetes—that is every other person in America! Twenty five percent of diabetics and ninety percent of pre-diabetics are not yet diagnosed. Caring for them will cost $3.4 trillion over the next 10 years. One in three Medicare dollars is spent on treating diabetes. Read those statistics again to let this really sink in. This is a global problem. From 1983 to 2011 world-wide diabetes increased from 35 million to 366 million and is projected to grow to 552 million by 2030. We recommend you read these statistics again to really let it sink in that our current approach is causing us to get sicker. We'll say that again—our current approach to 'healthcare' is causing our entire country to get sicker. Why? Because our current health care system is a 'Disease Centered Approach' instead of 'Personalized Health' which is a more 'patient centered' approach. A 'Disease Centered' system uses the same approach with everyone by classifying a disease. Your diagnosis of a particular 'disease' must follow the guidelines for a prescription of one or two medications for EVERYONE which won't resolve the root cause of your health issue because it is treating symptoms. We will get more into detail about this a little later, but for now we want you to understand the difference between 'Disease Centered' and 'Personalized Health' approaches to health care.

Take depression for example: When people become depressed, there are so many possible causes of their depression. It could be situational, such as losing a loved one, it could be nutritional in that they are lacking vital nutrients, it could also be hormonal or chemical. Yet conventional healthcare treats everyone's depression the same— they all get an antidepressant. But if there are several different possible causes for their depression, don't we need several different approaches to treatment? One person might need fish oil to help their brain work better chemically. Another might have a thyroid problem that needs an approach to restore hormone balance first (hormone replacement drugs should be the last, not the first step!). Another person's depression is caused by mercury toxicity and yet another might have low testosterone. By prescribing the same medication to all these different people, we ignore the root cause of their depression. They will be put on a medication for an indefinite amount of time, and if they try to go off of it, they will struggle because the cause still exists. They can take antidepressants, but if their toxicity isn't addressed or their testosterone level isn't restored for example, they won't ever recover.

Here's another way to think about it: Imagine that you have a sliver in your finger. How would you treat the painful sliver? The simple answer is to take the sliver out. You wouldn't just take pain medication to mask the symptom, right? But that's exactly how most doctors are trained to treat illness. Now imagine that you've got two slivers. Removing one doesn't solve the problem. You must find and remove ALL of them in order for the pain to go away and for healing to begin. In the same way, depression may be caused by low vitamin B12, thyroid dysfunction and inflammation for example—and of course we are not diagnosing here — but they all need to be fixed to begin to resolve the depression. Now you can begin to fully understand there are several different causes for a disease, therefore 'naming' a disease is almost worthless if you don't know the cause.

Doctors are encouraged to study which drug to prescribe for which disease; osteoporosis, diabetes, etc. - but that doesn't take the 'sliver' out of your hand and resolve the cause — if the 'sliver' was removed you wouldn't need the drugs. If you're just masking your pain, you may feel better for a while — but your disease process continues to ravage your body and will eventually catch up and manifest into a full blown, compromised life. If you have a stress fracture in your foot, you can take enough drugs to run a marathon — but your foot will be one heck of a lot worse after the race and now you need surgery. That's how disease is currently treated, with a 'Disease Centered' model, and that is why the rate of chronic disease is still rising in our country.

Insurance Covers Disease Centered Healthcare

Healthcare providers in the insurance medical system have a very specific compartment they are only allowed to work in to get paid by health insurance. They must follow the allopathic health model of symptom care, otherwise they will not get reimbursed and cannot continue doing business. The literal meaning of the word "Allopathic" is "to treat symptoms" so in this system, there is no effort to discover the underlying cause of your problem. Now, understand that we are not here to bash doctors. Most doctors have good intentions, but they are now handcuffed in an insurance-based system that does not allow them to spend the time needed, nor practice in a way that is truly patient centered.

Dr. Aseem Malhotra Cardiologist states "After almost two decades I have sadly come to the conclusion that honest doctors can no longer practice honest medicine. The healthcare system is corrupted, and no amount of money will fix it."

We're targeting the wrong things- high blood pressure, high cholesterol, and high blood sugar are NOT the cause of heart disease or diabetes. The culprit is what we eat, how much we exercise, manage our stress and environmental toxins. Lifestyle, environment and to a small extent genetics, influence your pathways to disease. Treating genetic risks is like blowing away the smoke while the fire rages on. Lifestyle and environment put the fires out. Unfortunately, insurance doesn't cover this approach because no one profits by this approach. It's not even part of medical education curriculum. Here's a disturbing fact that you may not know . . . The pharmaceutical industry is allowed to fund our medical schools. They begin romancing medical students in their first years and continue on throughout the student's medical school and internships. By the time these young doctors are ready to practice medicine, many of them are financially connected to the pharmaceutical companies. Think that might be a conflict of interest?

Most doctors do what they get paid to do- dispense medication and perform surgery. We hear so often from our wellness partners that the time spent with their doctor ranges from 8-10 minutes and they are sent on their way with another prescription for medication. We've heard the endless frustration, and we've witnessed the tears and heart wrenching stories from our people that have been through the mill, seen several doctors, but their health continues to decline. Maybe you know someone like this? Maybe this is your story. Doctors are trying their best, but insurance does not cover the time that must be spent with a patient to truly resolve the conditions. In addition, today's medical doctor receives no training in resolving the root cause of health issues. Doctors need to be paid to dispense education and lifestyle changes, some have a certain amount of education on the basics, but many do not. The National Council on Public Health developed policies to create a personalized health Regimen, but what's missing is the key ingredient- insurance payment! The future of healthcare is a personalized REGIMEN but the only way it will happen is if doctors are paid to do it. After being in practice a few years, doctors see the problems with just treating symptoms and they want better methods.

We need to rethink health care. When the collective cost of chronic disease is accounted for, it is the single biggest contributor to our national debt. **Seventy percent** of our federal budget is spent on Medicaid, Medicare and Social Security. The current system is unsustainable. Disease centered care uses the same approach with everyone. Every disease is treated with the same drug in the drug manual (PDR).

Examples (not prescribing)
- Suffering Arthritis? Take advil, alleve, celebrex, soma, flexaril—or worse, opioids.
- Depression? Prozac, Lexapro, Wellbutrin, and a long list of others.
- Osteoporosis? Fosamax.
- Can't sleep? Ambien.
- Allergies? Take Allegra or Zyrtec.
- Acid reflux? Prilosec, Prevacid or Maalox

This next statement may come as a surprise to you, but unfortunately most **natural or holistic approaches** follow the same disease—centered approach. Instead of a medication being prescribed, many 'Alternative' or 'Holistic' practitioners prescribe a nutrient or supplement. This is just trading one kind of pill for another. Yes, the side effects are not there with a supplement or nutrient but you are still not solving the root cause of the problem. You are still looking for a magic pill that does not exist.

Examples (not prescribing)

- Arthritis? MSM Methylsulfonylmethane Glucosamine
- Osteoporosis? Calcium and Vitamin D
- Insomnia? Valerian and Melatonin
- Heartburn? Licorice Root.
- Depression St. John's Wort.

Get Off The Conveyor Belt To Healthcare

It is our hope that the education contained in these pages can reach enough people, to not only help you and others adopt The Wellness Method to relieve suffering, but to create a tipping point where The Patient Centered Approach is commonplace and a first line of defense, instead of an alternative after everything else fails. No two people are alike. You are unique and have different requirements for creating, maintaining, and restoring your health. To find optimal health, each of us must find for ourselves what exactly those requirements are. When you were created, your mold was thrown away- from the shape of your ears, your physique, the curve of your neck, the color of your eyes and hair - you are individual and unique. It is true that as humans we do have some important things in common - for instance, we all have the need for fats, proteins and carbohydrates for health but each of us is biochemically unique and we differ in our ability to digest, assimilate and metabolize food. We all have enzymes and hormones that run the systems of our bodies, but we differ in the chemistry of those enzymes and hormones that will affect our needs to reach optimal health. Yes, it is possible for you to do this! We are addressing each person's unique biochemistry every day in our clinic.

CASE STUDY—Our Personalized Health Regimen From The Notes Of Dr. Kobsar

Case 1 Patricia- Osteoporosis

Patricia was a 57 year-old female who contacted me for severe osteoporosis. She had a T-score (the measurement for osteoporosis) of -4.90 (anything more than -2.5 is considered osteoporosis). Through her insurance-based care, she was prescribed Fosamax, Calcium and Vitamin D (symptom centered approach.) I ordered a comprehensive red blood cell mineral test and an assessment of her stomach lining which showed normal calcium but depleted magnesium and manganese due to poor absorption from stomach inflammation. It doesn't matter how organic the food is from the farmers market or how many vitamin supplements you take, if your stomach is not working it's just passing through. I created a 'Patient Centered Regimen' starting with improved absorption to really make an impact on her magnesium and manganese levels. Three months later, Patricia re-tested for osteoporosis. To her doctor's surprise, her T-score plummeted to -1.2 with *no sign of osteoporosis.* This happens all the time with our Personalized Health Regimens. If Patricia followed the disease centered approach to treat symptoms, it is debatable if she could have achieved these results. This Personalized Health Regimen offers a logical treatment approach based on your specific problem to correct system malfunctions and restore your health.

Your Personalized Health Regimen

Patricia mirrors many people who suffer needlessly when the underlying cause of the problem is overlooked. The Wellness Method is the future of healthcare in a personalized program rather than treating symptoms with a "one-size fits all" approach. Considering most of our mainstream media advertising promotes a disease-centered approach, it's unlikely that anytime soon you will hear about the benefits of a **Personalized Health Regimen** from those sources so, it is important for you to do your own research into this growing field. Our book will provide a good step into the field of Patient Centered Care that can help many suffering from fibromyalgia, arthritis, heart disease, allergies, and many other illnesses.

Another name we've already introduced you to is "Functional Medicine", which is a term we use frequently throughout this book. Now that you understand what Patient Centered Care is, it is an easy jump to understanding that Functional Medicine is the practice that focuses on improving the function of the body as a whole by resolving the root cause of health issues in each individual. No more guessing. No more experimenting. Its time you, and everyone for that matter are given the opportunity to have a program that is specific for you. Unfortunately, through this book, we can't do lab tests and read your reports but, we can get you on your way to becoming your healthiest you by educating you on this approach and providing you with clear action steps that will bring immediate results.

A Regimen Needs Baselines

We don't like to work in the dark and we highly suggest that you make sure that your current healthcare provider is not working in the dark. *"TEST! DON'T GUESS!"* is a phrase we live by. Before we put together a regimen for our partner's health, we need to have a clear understanding of what is going on, and even though we are frequently right about our assumptions, even after working in this method for 23 years, there are many times issues present themselves that we did not anticipate. Therefore, we always start with a complete a panel of tests to identify your current health status so that we can help you reach the outcomes you are looking for with your health. You can find a list of a few of the baseline tests we order before putting a program together by going to our website and becoming a member of our community. www.mywellnessmethod.com

ACTION STEPS

Throughout this book, you will be given Action Steps to help you begin to make small moves towards improving your health.

A Community of Health and Healing

We want to invite you to join the Wellness Method Community. It's an incredibly valuable resource where you can find additional online education and tools. Once you are registered, simply login and select from the many available resources and relevant content. If you are already a member, just login. Here's our website to get started: www.mywellnessmethod.com

Today's Action Steps

1. On our website, navigate to"Available Quizzes" and choose the "Health Quiz."
If you are already a member of Wellness Method Community, just login and follow the link to Available Quizzes.

2. Do your homework. You may need to do some research if you are struggling with a health issue or disease. Good resources include government and organization websites that end in ".gov" or ".org."

3. Enlist your doctor. Ask him or her to help you go beyond your symptoms by ordering tests that can help identify root problems. Remember there are ways to find the cause—almost all diseases have a few fundamental causes- namely toxins, infections, allergens, diet, lifestyle, and stress. Be a detective.

4. Consider finding an expert. You may have to search for a doctor who can think differently and address the causes of disease. Some doctors have now been trained in functional medicine and have adopted a new way of thinking about health that addresses the individual genetic, environmental, and lifestyle causes of disease.

5. Read up. Learn so you can advocate for yourself when you speak to your healthcare practitioners.

EDUCATION

Regimen
Educational Curriculum
Coaching
Reducing Inflammation
Endocrine System
Alignment of Your Structure
Total Nutrition
Exercise

"The greatest enemy of knowledge is not ignorance, it is the illusion of knowledge.

~ Stephen Hawking

Remember the days when we all had encyclopedias on our bookshelf? Ok we might be 'dating' ourselves here, but we want to make a point: They were a staple item in many homes and they were impressive to look at because we all knew that within the pages was a massive amount of knowledge. In some homes the covers were worn, pages torn, food and coffee stains muddled the pages. In other homes they were shiny and new because they were rarely, if ever used. So, let us ask you: The books that sat on the shelves, unused, shiny and new . . . did they make difference in the lives of those that lived in that home? Obviously, the answer is no. The books are 'education', however that education was never used.

We all know the phrase "Knowledge Is Power," right? But is it really? Think about it - we have a massive amount of information at our fingertips on our phones, computers and now on some watches! Everyone has access to all that 'knowledge' so everyone should be powerful right? Well, we know that is not true so clearly knowledge is not power. It only becomes powerful when you use it. Knowledge has no value unless you put it into practice in your life. Then you own it, then its embedded in your life. That is where your power lies. There is a lot of generic advice being dispensed in the media by healthcare providers, fitness enthusiasts and celebrities. Just go spend a few minutes on Facebook. Everyone is a specialist and while many of them mean well we always say there are three kinds of information;

- misinformation
- bad information
- good information that does not apply to you.

> "Information is useless if its not put into action and applied to your life."
>
> ~ Judy Pearson Kobsar

If you want to have true freedom, if you want to be **independent of medications and minimize your dependence on doctors and the health insurance system, you must 'learn' how to take control of your health and then act on it.** Our goal with this book is to give you a solid, comprehensive foundation to teach you the principles of our system that work, and then encourage you to find a health care provider that practices functional medicine. Whether it be us or someone else, we want you to have support in your journey and have an expert create your Personalized Health Regimen. With the combination of what you learn here and the guidance of a qualified practitioner, you will own your health. Your life depends on it!

How And Where Did Conventional Medicine Go Wrong?

Indigenous cultures worldwide have long been known to honor the mind/body/environment connection. So why did Western Medicine embrace the opposite view? Blame it on Rene Descartes, a 17th century French philosopher ("I think, therefore I am"). Descartes needed human bodies for dissection studies and he made a deal with the Pope of his era. He would leave the soul, the mind and the emotions under the Church's jurisdiction, and modern medicine would only take the physical body as its domain, thus dividing the human being into two separate parts that were not to overlap. According to this paradigm, to understand humans, all we had to do was take the body apart and study the parts. And so, the foundation was laid for hundreds of years of relating health and disease exclusively to treating the physical body. Thankfully, this theory is slowly changing.

When we work with our wellness partners, the Education Principle is a substantial part of their curriculum. We fill them up with life giving wisdom about their health and the systems of their body. They are given books to read, videos to watch, lifestyle changes to practice, classes to attend and they receive a lot of one on one support from our team. Our goal is for them to 'own' their health so they can become empowered by it and in turn pass it on to their loved ones. In this book, our goal is to educate you, the reader, about more than just your health. Our goal is to educate you about our current healthcare system so that you understand the bigger picture and how it may have affected you and those you love. And we are going to shoot straight and tell it like it is, with no filter, because it's time. It's time for the public to be educated on the underlying root cause of why our healthcare system is causing our country to become more dependent on medications than ever before. And it's time for you to understand what lifestyle choices are causing our society to be sicker than we've ever been before. Our intention is to be messengers of the truth, but you must be willing to accept it as so.

What Did Galileo Know About Health?

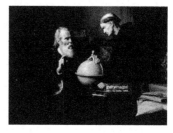

Galileo's claim to fame may not have been the secrets to beating cancer, but his story represents how we look at changes in our belief system. Before you read any further, ask yourself- "How do I react upon discovering a truth that violates my current beliefs?" Imagine yourself at a time when we believed that the world was flat. You "knew" the world was flat, as did everyone around you. Furthermore, all the reputable leaders; presidents and governors, religious leaders, scientists and teachers, all believed the fact that the world was flat. How would a rational, thinking individual, respond when Galileo comes along with proof that not only is the earth round, but it revolves around the sun? If you are a rational person engaged in the pursuit of truth, then you are happy to get to learn this new reality. If, however, you are a fearful person and easily influenced by "authority," which is the majority of our society, then you are more likely to react to the new statement with ridicule and doubt and sometimes even with hostility.

What Happened To Galileo?

One of the most brilliant and innovative scientists ever known was in prison during what should have been the most productive years of his life. He had shattered the myths of his day by stating new truths. When Galileo proposed that a small stone and a big stone would fall at the same speed the ignorant masses and all the scientific authorities of the day laughed at such a notion. When Galileo dropped his big stone and little stones from the top of the Tower of Pisa, and to everyone's astonishment they hit the ground at precisely the same instant, an amazing number of people went into total denial when faced with this new truth. They presumed Galileo somehow tricked them. When Galileo proved that the earth rotated around the sun, the establishment was so threatened that denial was not enough, so they locked up 'this fanatic' and put him away! We scoff at this now but has anything changed today?

The belief system surrounding health care is flawed. Many people are following a system that has obviously failed and has been failing for a very long time. And all the money spent on healthcare does nothing to change our results. Yes, we live longer, but how is the quality of that 'long life?' Some say that "we don't live longer, we die longer". The USA has the most expensive healthcare system in the world and yet we are rated #72 by the World Health Organization on overall health and #51 on life expectancy. Third world countries like Cuba are ranked higher than America!

It's been said that "The greatest obstacle to discovering the shape of the earth, was not ignorance, but the illusion of knowledge." The same can be said for healthcare. What we think we know about disease isn't working. Anyone that is paying attention can see it and we are waking up to that fact. Some third world country's healthcare systems are outperforming the most expensive system in the world, the American healthcare system. That's why we are at a crossroads, where the old ideas we have about disease have less meaning as we understand more about the importance of individual differences in determining illness and bringing resolutions. In fact, we are at a time in healthcare where the old ideas are rapidly becoming obsolete. The new healthcare says the world is round, while the old healthcare says the world is flat. It's clear where we're headed. This is a time when personalized healthcare will replace symptom-based diagnosis and disease. It's a very exciting time and we are thrilled that you are now a part of this transformation!

This is your last chance. After this there is no turning back. You take the blue pill, the story ends. You wake up in your bed and believe whatever you want to. You take the red pill, you stay in Wonderland, and I show you how deep the rabbit hole goes. Remember, all I'm offering is the truth. Nothing more.

~ Morpheus, the Matrix Film, 1999

Are You Engaged In The Pursuit Of Truth, Or In Clinging To Popular Belief Systems?

The contents of this book are based on scientific facts, not 'our opinions'. Your ability to successfully Recreate your health is highly dependent on your emotional attachment to a system that does not produce results. As someone so eloquently put it: *"The definition of insanity is doing the same thing over and over and expecting different results."* So where will you stand? Are you clinging to the popular belief system, or are you in pursuit of the truth? If your answer is . . . The Pursuit of Truth, then we can say with a high degree of certainty that you will enjoy the road less traveled and join the growing number of exceptional people who have decided to follow this proven path to optimal health.

We understand your next question might be, "Why didn't I know about this approach before?". So to help you understand why you may not have known what optimal health really is, we want to bust a couple of popular myths for you throughout this book. We call them "Big Fat Lies", and here's one:

BIG FAT LIE: We get fat and *then* sick,

Fact: We were *already* sick- that's WHY we got fat. Your body responds to sickness by holding on to fat.

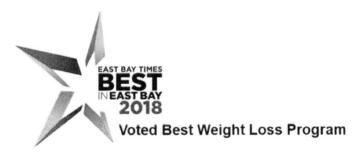

Voted Best Weight Loss Program

We were shocked the first time we won an award for the best weight loss program because we are not a weight loss clinic, we are a Functional Medicine Clinic. When you restore your health, your body no longer needs to hold on to fat and it will release it. It doesn't matter how many hours you exercise or how much you limit the calories you eat- if you are not healthy your body will hold on to fat. Our focus is to restore your health first and foremost, and when that happens everything else follows. This is where the new 'mind set' comes in.

"Health Gain = Weight Loss"

~ Judy Pearson Kobsar

The one requirement that is necessary for you to benefit from the information in this book is an open mind to create your **"Mind Shift"** about the effects of food, exercise and your health. Here's the truth- being overweight is a 'symptom' of sickness, it's a wakeup call that things are going wrong in your body. Excess fat is a warning sign that your health is faltering. Your body is sending you a message to listen! Hypertension, high cholesterol, high blood pressure- these all go hand in hand with weight gain for a reason. Your body wants you to make a change- and it's NOT asking you to put medication in your body.

"Education sets you free, but only if you use it!"

~ Dr. Bradley Kobsar

Disease appears real just as the earth appeared flat. In a book called "Disease Delusion", Dr. Jeffrey Bland shatters the concept of disease. Over the past 30 years Dr. Bland has contributed more to medical science and functional medicine than anyone. He found that disease does not exist in the way we think about it. Doctors use the disease names to match to a medication, but not to learn the root cause of the problem. Consider the patient who feels sad, hopeless, loss of libido, isolated and no appetite. Does naming their condition, "Depression" change anything for the patient? Does it help in any way? Depressed is simply the name given to people who happen to share similar symptoms. It is then treated with an anti-depressant which research studies report that it works only a little better than chance. The causes of the same symptoms, for all the people with the same "disease," differ immensely. In fact, the underlying cause of depression can arise from many different possibilities. Examples (not prescribing):

- A diet high in tuna that caused mercury toxicity
- A diet low in omega-3 fatty acids deficiency
- A high-sugar diet that has caused pre-diabetes.
- Antibiotics that have altered the normal stomach bacteria, which altered brain chemistry.
- A leaky gut that activates the immune system, producing antibodies against the thyroid leading to low thyroid function.
- Years of drugs for acid reflux that cause vitamin B12 deficiency
- A gene called MTHFR that leads to folate deficiency
- Vitamin D deficiency

Diet, environment, lifestyle, all create different imbalances, yet all can cause depression. As students of Wellness and Functional Medicine for over twenty years, we witness daily both the failures of our current healthcare and the miracles of the new healthcare paradigm. Wellness Medicine is not simply about improving diet, exercise, managing stress and environmental toxins, it is a personalized method of getting to the root cause and restoring balance. Above all, it is the science of 'creating health'. If we do that, disease often goes away as a side effect of creating health. Paradigm shifts are hard and there are plenty of detractors, yet the evidence is here. The failure of our current approach is evident to any student of health care and the time is ripe for a major shift. We have the power to end needless suffering for millions of people. Every doctor, every healthcare insurer, every hospital and every government leader involved in making health policies has the power, but unfortunately, all the stakeholders are heavily invested in the current system. And making changes will result in lost time and losses in their investments, which are so large that our American economy will feel the effects.

The 3 Worst Things Your Doctor Can Tell You

Sometimes doctors tell patients things that cause them to feel defeated and depressed because they totally take away their power to help themselves. It takes them out at the knees and creates a passive victim just waiting for something to happen. Here are the three worst things that doctors tell their patient; The reason for the symptoms you are experiencing is because of . . .

1. Genetics
2. Arthritis
3. Age

When doctors tell you this, they are in fact telling you that you can't do anything to help your problem and that you are just a victim of your circumstances. But NOTHING could be FURTHER FROM

THE TRUTH! The problem is that you have been accepting a slowly diminishing quality of life for years, maybe even decades- because you didn't think you had any other choice, but you do!

1. Genetics

"Here is the amazing thing about Genetics: You can take a stem cell and put it in a petri dish in a certain chemistry for it to live in and it becomes a muscle cell. You can change the chemistry of the culture medium of that same cell and it becomes a bone cell. Change it again and it becomes a fat cell. Genetically it remains the same, but the environment was changed. This research is repeatable all day, everyday, all day long! You can also change the environment of your cells with the choices you make with how you live your life. The caterpillar and the butterfly have the exact same DNA. They are the same organism but are receiving and responding to a different organizing signal." Bruce Lipton PhD

The genes that define your physical attributes cannot be changed. If you have blue eyes, you cannot change that. Disease processes and genes operate differently in that multiple genes must get 'switched on' to afflict your body and cause internal change. Cancer needs at least 12 different genes to get switched on to become active, yet we hear people often say, "I have bad genes." We also hear, "My dad had diabetes, its genetic, so that's why I have diabetes." We would like to now shed light on this for you.

From 1983 to 2008, the number of diabetics in the world increased nearly seven times, from 35 million to 240 million. It is impossible that genetics caused this increase in such a short amount of time. Human gene codes only change 0.2 percent every 20,000 years but our lifestyle and environment has radically changed in the last 100 years. A search for a diabetes gene or magic pill has led us nowhere but what researchers have found is that the major cause is not genetics. Today we know that genetics only factors between 3% to

9% of your overall health. 95% comes from your life choices that in turn SWITCH ON your genes, to get expressed under the conditions that we give them.

It's Not My Fault, It's My Genes!

We want to tell you here and now, do not just accept that you were handed the fat genes, or the diabetes genes. There are 32 genes that are associated with obesity in the general population and they only account for 9% of obesity. So even if you had all 32 genes which is close to impossible you would only put on 22 pounds. By the year 2050 its projected 50% of all Americans will be obese- up from the current 35%. But our genes don't change that fast- what has changed is the amount of sugar we consume. We went from eating 10 pounds of sugar every year per person in the 1800's, to 152 pounds per person per year today! Now throw in another 146 pounds of flour per year which turns into sugar inside the body, and at these doses they have the same effect as taking drugs, highjacking our metabolism making us store fat and making us sick.

The truth is that obesity is caused by many factors and genetics plays a very small and insignificant role. Where were all the fat people 100 years ago? The fact is they didn't exist except on very rare occasions. We all have genetic risks but do we all express them? No, but we get to decide if they are expressed. Genes are just a blueprint, but we are the architects of our health.

How we eat, how we exercise, how we manage stress and environmental toxins all effect our gene expression. In 2010 a groundbreaking study found that **90% of disease is due to environment, not genes as reported in the journal 'Science.'** Air, water, diet, drugs, pollutants, heavy metals, radiation, physical and emotional stressors all create inflammation, therefore the genetic code doesn't change, but gene expression does. This is very powerful! We turn our genes on or off by the way we live, this is called **Epigenetics**. If your grandmother smoked, ate too much sugar, or was exposed to lead, she may have "turned on" genes that lead to diabetes but you have the power to change your gene expression. You can chart a new course for your DNA to "turn off" the genes your grandmother "turned on".

2. Arthritis

Telling someone "you have arthritis" is like telling them, you have joints and muscles . . . because 95% of arthritis is from joint degeneration and NO ONE ESCAPES this life without having any wear and tear on their joints. That's like expecting the tires on your car to last forever. We all have wear and tear but, we all don't have pain and swelling. So, if we all have it why do some people have severe pain and even disability while others just cruise right through life? Dr. Kobsar has had bone spurs in his neck since he was in his 20's from years of playing ice hockey and yet has little pain or stiffness. 'How can that be?' It's simple really, take care of your body and your body will take care of you. You can bet that if he had unrelenting, chronic neck pain and went to see the doctor, he would be sent for an X-ray and referred for an MRI and a surgical consultation. Many surgeons would put his X-ray or MRI films up on lighted view box and most likely proceed to talk about how the bone spurs require surgery. They may use terms and phrases like "bone on bone" and 'disabled' in 10 or 20 years . . . . They may even say there is a chance of becoming paralyzed. Now, certainly not every surgeon does this, but many do.

3. Age

"There's no reason why your 20's should be your peak years. Your Metabolic Age can stay in your 20's for three, four or five decades! But in order to live that way, you must stop making the mistakes that cause premature aging. These repeated mistakes will eventually make damage recovery and rejuvenation impossible and we don't like to see that happen."

~ Dr. Bradley Kobsar

We hear so often from our Wellness Partners that their doctor told them, "Well, you are getting older, and these things just begin to happen." We all age but are we all disabled because of our age? Is everyone sick once they hit a certain age? Of course not. We don't expect every doctor to have all the answers, we certainly don't. But we will admit if we can't figure it out, we will refer you to another healthcare provider that can figure it out.

Things change as we age. We know that muscles atrophy, hormones decline, neurotransmitters decrease, etc. . . . So, it's important to get tested to know where you stand so that you can get the right treatment to have a positive effect. We can test to see if your chronological age (actual years) compares to your 'Metabolic Age', which is a critical baseline measure that we track as you move through your program. Our goal is to help you grow younger metabolically. You CAN achieve metabolic youth by following the principles outlined in this book and get started right away. If not now, when?

3 Reasons for Accelerated Metabolic Aging

1. **Hormones and Neurotransmitters.** Neurotransmitters are like hormones in the brain in that they provide chemical messages. These are often overlooked yet are common reasons for weight gain and disease. They will be addressed on a deeper level in the chapter on the Endocrine Principal.

2. **Food:** One of the most important causes of a slow metabolism is not eating enough, yes, you read that correctly—not eating enough can cause your metabolism to slow down. Not eating enough of the right kind of foods also contributes to a sluggish metabolism. We are the first generation that must put a high priority on understanding how genetically modified foods, processed foods, trans fats and sugar (especially high fructose corn syrup), are affecting our metabolism due to the pervasiveness of them in our food supply.

3. **Muscle Loss:** Experts agree that muscles not only have the ability to 'slow' the aging process, but they can even **reverse it** given the right circumstances! Healthy muscle mass is essential, the more of it you have the greater your metabolic rate. More muscle means less problems with your blood sugars and fat accumulation. Conditioned muscles keep you mobile and independent. We are not talking about the excessive muscle mass you see in bodybuilder magazines, we are really just talking about you maintaining the muscle you have and making it more efficient. In fact, adding a couple of pounds of muscle will supercharge your metabolism giving you the ability to burn more calories every day. You see, you're losing about one percent of your muscle every year after age 30 unless you do something to reverse that process. In the following chapters you will learn how to efficiently wake up that dormant muscle and add a few pounds of this metabolically active fat burning tissue. **Building a pound of muscle is very, very 'metabolically expensive' and that is a very good thing! The body has to burn 45,000 calories to build a pound of muscle.** Where are all of these extra calories going to be found every day to meet your metabolic needs? From your fat cells . . . that's right, they are a ready and available source of energy. This is why you want to add 3 or 4 pounds of muscle- muscle that you won't even notice in the size of your body, as it is much more dense than fat.

Conventional Allopathic Medicine Misses the Fundamental Laws of Biology

Allopathic, insurance based medicine treats disease with medication or surgery. That's what it is designed to do, and when it comes to emergency interventions it is still the best medicine in the world. If you've ever been in a car accident or had a finger cut off, there is no place better to be than in an emergency room in the USA.

Conventional medicine has amazing emergency room doctors and the high tech medical equipment to treat these situations. But those types of accidents make up less than 10% of healthcare. When it comes to the other 90%, which is chronic illness, this approach simply doesn't work. As proof, in 1991, the prestigious British Medical Journal reported that 85% of all medical procedures and surgeries are scientifically unproven. This was confirmed by the World Health Organization report that 90% of all diseases prevalent today are not treatable with orthodox medical procedures. The United States is ranked 47th among all developed countries in the treatment of chronic disease even though we spend more than the majority of other countries on the treatment of chronic disease.

For example, when it comes to diabetes most doctors just follow blood sugar, which actually rises very late in the disease process. If your blood sugar is 125, you don't have diabetes but if it's over 126 you now have diabetes because someone arbitrarily decided this- and they do nothing to help treat impending problems. Daren was a Wellness Partner who came to us with mildly elevated blood sugar. We asked Daren if he had seen his doctor about this. He said yes. We then inquired, "What did your doctor say?" Daren's doctor had told him, "We are going to wait and watch until your blood sugar is more elevated, and then we are going to treat you with medication for diabetes." This attitude is absurd and harmful in the face of what we know about the problems that occurs even in the early stages of diabetes. Science is now showing us that many people with pre-diabetes never get diabetes, but they are at severe risk just the same. Pre-diabetes isn't PRE-anything, it's a serious health condition and needs to be treated as early as possible.

More to the point, this approach completely ignores more subtle clues from symptoms and signs of disease, which may highlight underlying metabolic imbalances (especially when complemented by further testing). These imbalances may be remedied by the appropriate treatment—treatment that is not focused on some disease, but instead works to remove those things that alter or damage our functioning, and provides those things that enhance, optimize, and normalize our functioning by balancing the system rather than treating the symptom. We need to treat the system, not the symptom; the patient, not the disease.

Are we harping on this point? Yes! And we will continue to do so until we hit a critical mass, a tipping point so that this line of thinking becomes the norm instead of 'the alternative'. We must first 'undo' what's been done to the mindset of Americans when it comes to the definition of healthcare. And we understand that in order to truly EDUCATE, we must unwind the magic pill mentality first, clear it out and provide scientifically sound, proven points to reshape our thinking around what true care of our health means.

We are not talking about alternative medicine here. This is a science-based, fundamental change in our way of thinking about health and disease. The treatments are grounded in nutrition and lifestyle, complemented by the interaction between your genetics and environmental factors.

We keep up with the growing number of requests for appointments that come into our practice, and seeing our Wellness Partners is the heart and soul of our work- but we have found that we must also make time to change the healthcare paradigm through research, professional education, and writing so we can help reach more people. We created an online program for our approach and revised our website to serve more people all across the country. It's been an amazing journey and we are just getting started! More importantly, we have found the right people to help support this work and by working together and supporting each other we are able to give our wellness partners the best care by staying on top of the latest research. We work closely as a team to help everyone recreate their health.

Prescription Drugs:
#1 Cause Of Fatal Overdoses In America

Today's drug users are not out on the streets causing mayhem, they are inside, mostly alone and quiet. They are altered, depressed and often unbalanced enough to pick up a gun and cause widespread devastation to quiet communities. And they are many times doing damage to themselves. Overdose deaths are often obscured by coroners' reports to hide what is happening. When the cause of death is inescapable - young bodies found in bedrooms or fast-food restrooms - it is often, too shameful to share. Parents of dead teenagers are unlikely to publicize their agony. The old stereotype of a heroin junkie as a dropout or hippie has disappeared, especially in high schools. Athletes are given opioids to mask injuries to keep them on the field which they shared with cheerleaders and other peers and because of their social status, they have rebranded our perception of drug addicts. Now opiate addicts come wrapped in some of the most promising, physically fit, and capable young men and women of our generation. Often it is under the discretion of their doctors and coaches. It is not intentional. Coaches, parents and doctors do not intend to harm young people.

Most doctors have good intentions and desperately want to help their patients, but unfortunately, they are handcuffed in an insurance-based health and pharmaceutical system that takes away their freedom to practice medicine the way they want to. In addition, drug companies are not policed by the Food and Drug Administration (FDA) the way they should be. A drug should be proven both effective and safe

BEFORE it is prescribed to millions of people. Sadly, that is often not the case. When a drug company performs a study, ALL the results must be submitted to the FDA. But, many pharmaceutical companies ONLY submit the data they want published in medical journals. That means that negative studies are being hidden. And when drug studies are sponsored by drug companies—as most are—they find positive outcomes at 4 times the rate of independently funded studies.

Prescribed medication overdoses kill more than cocaine and heroin overdoses combined. At what point does massive deaths provoke a government response? Imagine a terror attack that killed over 40,000 people or a virus that threatened to kill 52,000 Americans this year. Wouldn't any government make this a top national priority? Vibrant good health is a universal objective, but in America, few people have the opportunity to experience it. We are committed to changing that. We are committed to helping you reach optimal health by identifying underlying causes of disease and chronic pain, both of which are resolved with diet and lifestyle modifications. Our goal is to help you create wellness using a natural but comprehensive approach to health. Our wish is to have everyone say, "I didn't know I could feel this good!" Because we treat the person, not the disease, and because we work on the core systems of the body to get healthier and this can help improve any condition.

More Education: How The Cholesterol Story Started

In 1961, Ancel Keys changed the diet of our entire country. He told us that saturated fat raised cholesterol in our body and that created heart disease. He was the originator of the cholesterol theory- and what was his expertise that gave him the authority to do this? Well, he had a BA in economics and a PhD in Fish physiology! We ignored all the other scientists including a major study in 1957 in the Journal of the American Medical Association that looked at all the diet studies and found that a high protein, high fat and low carbohydrate diet was the best way to lose weight. We ignored everyone else because Ancel Keys was on the cover of Time Magazine. We now know that Keys hid some of his research to make it fit his theory. He misled everyone by slightly distorting his data on saturated fat and the result is that Americans have been stuck in his dogma, getting sicker, fatter and depressed for the past 60 years.

How Fat Was Demonized and Sugar Was Left Untouched

We have known about the problems of sugar for long time. Back in the 1960s there was a battle going on between sugar and fat. We decided to leave sugar alone and pointed at fat as the bad guy and that has shaped health policy in America for the last 50 years. It was all a fraud. Christine Kearns reported in the Journal of the American Medical Association in 2016 that while she was digging through boxes of letters in the basement of a Harvard library she found history on a trade group called the Sugar Research Foundation. This group was trying to influence public understanding of sugar's role in disease and paid off two famous Harvard school of public health scientists, Dr. Fredrick Stare and his assistant Mark Hegsted,(who later became head of the USDA). These two exonerated sugar as the problem and got paid $6500 in 1967, which would be equivalent to about $50,000 today. The sugar industry funding was not disclosed, and consumption of sugar grew exponentially over the past 50 years along with sickness and suffering in our population. (Excerpt from Robert Lustig MD, PhD)

The Truth About Statins

Doctors have been taught that cholesterol is the cause of heart attacks even though half of all people who have heart attacks have NORMAL cholesterol levels. So, your doctor frequently prescribes statins like Lipitor and Zocor to lower cholesterol and reduce the risk of heart attacks, however, here's what is proven: The reason statins lower the risk of heart attacks is NOT because they lower cholesterol, but because they lower inflammation. Dr. Paul Ridker of Harvard performed a study that showed the risk of heart attacks was only reduced if inflammation was lowered and LDL cholesterol was lowered—but not if LDL cholesterol was lowered alone.

(2) Inflammation Reduction Cuts Risk Of Heart Attack, Stroke. November 14, 2002. N Engl J Med 2002; 347: 1557-1565.

Opioids: America's Deadliest Drug Overdose Crisis.

The American people consume 99% of the world's hydrocodone and 81% of its oxycodone. Opium, morphine, fentanyl, heroine, etc., have hooked more than 2 million of us and claimed more American lives last year than we lost in the Vietnam War. The poppy is now responsible for a decline in the life spans in America for two years in a row, a decline that isn't happening in any other developed nation. The spread of fentanyl can be thought of as a mass poisoning. Think back to the poison discovered in a handful of tainted Tylenol pills in 1982. Every bottle of Tylenol in America was immediately recalled; in Chicago, police went into neighborhoods with loudspeakers to warn residents of the danger. That was in response to a scare that killed, in total, seven people. In 2016, 20,000 people died from overdosing on opioids.

Proof: Opioids Are No Better Than Other Medications For Chronic Pain

A first-of-its-kind study in the Journal of the American Medical Association compared opioids to non-opioid drugs in patients with back pain or hip or knee arthritis. As of 2016, 67 prescriptions were being written for every 100 Americans. The same year, there were 14,500 opioid-related deaths. All this time, doctors and patients have been operating with no high-quality evidence for opioids over the long term. Finally, a high-quality randomized controlled trial was published showing opioids work no better than non-opioids thanks to Dr. Erin Krebs, at the Minneapolis VA Center. Dr. Krebs answered the question, 'Do opioids help patients with chronic pain in the long run?' Answer- A resounding "NO". Krebs compared chronic pain patients on opioids (morphine, hydrocodone, and oxycodone) to patients on non-opioids (Tylenol, naproxen, or meloxicam), measuring their pain and function over a year. Patients on opioids did no better than those not taking opioids. In fact, opioid takers even reported being in more pain so it's not just that opioids were not better — they were worse! It's become clear through numerous studies that America's opioid epidemic has been fueled by heavy marketing of the pharmaceutical companies

"Evidence-Based" Medicine

The Evidence-Based approach in the insurance-based healthcare system is considered the highest standard of care with the idea that we make decisions based on sound medical evidence. It's a good in theory, but it only works if that evidence can be trusted to find the best treatment. This model fails if the motive is profit. Unfortunately, in our healthcare system, business trumps science. In 2004, the National Institute of Health's National Cholesterol Education Program, dramatically lowered the ideal "bad" or LDL cholesterol level. This led to guidelines that expanded the number of Americans who "should" take statin drugs from 13 million to 36 million. It is reported that eight of the nine panel members who established these new guidelines had industry ties. An independent group of over 30 scientists in a letter to the National Institutes of Health publicly opposed these recommendations.

Why this matters to you

We shared the education in this chapter with you so that you understand 'research' and advertisements are flawed and can cause great harm. Our intent is to educate you about the other side of the story. Important points about research to remember:

1. What gets studied depends on who is funding it. Since drug companies fund most of the research, other therapies that work better—such as lifestyle or nutritional therapies—get very little, if any, funding for research studies.
2. Drug companies are aided by the FDA, which studies prove, suppresses and the negative pharmaceutical research, but they do however publicize the positive studies. This leads doctors to think they have all the evidence when the reality is they don't.
3. Doctors, patients, and the media believe they have the whole truth, often until it is too late, like with Zetia, Premarin Estrogen and Vioxx- those were 'popular' drugs that eventually were exposed and had successful lawsuits brought against them. The evidence was there, but no one looked at or publicized it. This makes it very difficult for consumers to get the best treatments for their health and the whole truth about drugs.

Ok, that was a lot of disturbing evidence but our main purpose for this chapter is to educate you and our main goal with this book is to open your eyes to what's beyond the advertisements you see and hear every day.

How to Protect Yourself

1. Follow the money! Research the new "miracle drug" in the news. Learn who funded the study and any Big Pharma affiliations of the authors.

2. Don't assume that drugs are the answer. Heart disease is NOT a deficiency of statins; pain is NOT a deficiency of opioids. Look at how your lifestyle interacts with your genes.

3. Learn to search for answers by using PUBMED (the National Library of Medicine) to review what other research studies say. Adapt the motto used at University of California San Francisco, ***"In God We Trust, Everyone Else Has to Show Their Research Data"***.

4. Write your Congressmen to demand new regulations to protect us:
    - Make it illegal for Big Pharma to design research studies or interpret results.
    - Limit their lobbyists ability to influence government.
    - Demand a government policy to prevent former drug company executives from working at the FDA.

5. Assess your lifestyle and environmental factors. This is the basis of the Wellness Method's success with chronic illness as it treats the underlying cause of your problem.

6. Drugs are a backup when needed but take a long hard look at the research data on those drugs. You might be surprised by what you find. You can stay informed by visiting https: //www.drugwatch.com/ to know which drugs and drug companies are being sued.

Why Is Education Important?

You can see now why knowing how the healthcare industry works is important to restoring your health. Now you know how to begin making informed decisions for yourself. It's your body, it's your life—the more you know, the more power you have to make the right decisions and start taking action in the right direction. Remember, knowledge is NOT power until you act on what you've learned. Then you own it and you are in control!

Our goal is to not only educate you about the healthcare system but to teach you about the new paradigm of functional medicine, and also about your body. Our intent here is to give you as many points as we can to get you started on your path to health. It's important for you to understand that not everything you read, even in the 'most respected' medical journals and studies, is going to have a bias, and its not always true. Often there is an alternative agenda. What might that agenda be? You guessed it- money. So beware, follow the money and filter out the articles and studies that have a 'spin' on them to benefit big business.

ACTION STEPS:

Education sets you Free! Along with educational materials we provided throughout the book, here is a web link that lets you view most of these movies streaming online for free. **http://www.sprword. com/health.html**

Watch. Enjoy. Learn. Forever.

If by any chance the site is taken down, or, is discontinued then refer to **Netflix.**

- **Fed UP** Produced by Katy Couric, some great interviews with highly respected doctors.
- **Food Inc.** Crucial when it comes to understanding the food industry.
- **Bought** We are waking up to the fact that we don't have a private system, we have a pharmaceuticalized system and it has created the sickest species ever to inhabit this earth . . . our children. Your food, your health, your family's health has been Bought.

- **The Magic Pill** Doctors, scientists and chefs around the globe combat illness with dietary changes, believing fat should be embraced as a source of fuel.
- **Scientists Under Attack** The attack on scientists is very well structured by the biotech industry. Anywhere in the world, if someone finds a problem that can threaten this empire, they are jumped on.
- **Food Matters** This film examines how the food we eat can help or hurt our health.
- **Fat, Sick and Nearly Dead** Australian film maker attempts to take control of his health during a cross-country trek across America.
- **The Future of Food** They were allowed the patent a breast cancer gene so many researchers who were working to cure breast cancer were no longer allowed to research that gene unless they paid very, very high fees. Pharmaceutical companies have sued university researchers who were using 'their genes'. One of the most disturbing economic trends of our times."
- **Forks over Knives**
- **Supersize Me**

COACHING

Regimen
Educational Curriculum
Coaching
Reducing Inflammation
Endocrine System
Alignment of Your Structure
Total Nutrition
Exercise

The moment you change your perception is the moment you rewrite the chemistry of your body. Your cells do not question information sent by your nervous system. They respond equally to life-giving perceptions and self-destructive misperceptions. Consequently, our perceptions greatly influence the fate of our lives."

~ Bruce H. Lipton, PhD

A Note From Judy

Personal Growth is a term we hear often. But I want you to know that personal growth and spiritual growth go hand in hand and are necessary for change to become permanent. I have studied many forms of spirituality and have embarked on different personal growth paths. They all come back to the same two things:

1) You must change your mind to change your life and,
2) You must believe in something higher than yourself.

Changing your mind means growing personally, but in order to do that you must understand the higher power that exists. Whatever you want to call it- God, Source Energy, Spirit or the like—that higher power is there for you to tap into to facilitate a mind-shift and to grow spiritually. You cannot have one without the other. Changing your mind begins and ends with YOU. Your thoughts about yourself is where you must start and find your way into a belief of the Divine.

In all of my studies I've embraced a belief in in God, a Higher Power, my Maker, Source Energy and The Universe. I encourage you to find a belief system and make it work for you so that you continue to evolve yourself. Changing your mind is non-negotiable if you desire improvement in your health, finances, relationships- any aspect of your life quite frankly. But it takes a profound commitment to discipline your mind and a deep understanding of why we are here on this earth. I remember clearly in my 20's I had a constant nagging desire to know the meaning of life. I wanted to know why I was here on earth. Someone told me once that 'it is a test' . . . but that just didn't work for me because I kept wanting to know what was being tested and what was the outcome of 'the test'? If you passed, if you failed, what was the meaning of each? So, I wrestled with that for a while and then tossed it aside years later to continue my search.

Wallace Wattles, author of 'The Science of Being Great' states, "We are here to make the most of ourselves." As I studied his philosophy more, along with the rest of my spiritual and personal foundation, I understood that if we make the most of ourselves then it automatically translates to helping others make the most of themselves and that serves the greater good. THAT is where I finally rested in my belief of 'why we are here'—to make the most of ourselves. I saw it in action with others that were developing and evolving themselves. So, I went to work and used all of my spiritual beliefs to begin to make the most of myself, and I witnessed the manifestation of not only my evolution, but the evolution of my loved ones and those I affect in my life.

I tell this story because as Americans (and especially women, and most especially mothers) we tend to think that if we focus on ourselves and 'make the most of ourselves' . . . well that's a selfish thing. We are supposed to take care of everyone else, give to the needy, donate, put ourselves out for our children, our spouses and families. Yes we must care for our loved ones and make sacrifices, but I learned very quickly that going overboard on that only runs you into the ground and then you are no good for anyone. You begin to resent, get ill, carry the burden of exhaustion and lack of self-fulfillment. I know, I was there.

So in order to truly change your mind, you must first clear out your old beliefs about who you are. If your thoughts are negative towards yourself, if you condemn yourself, then that is a sign that you must change your beliefs about yourself. When you do that, your life will change, and you will discover what your purpose is. Everyone has a purpose. Not everyone's purpose is meant to change the world, but everyone's purpose is guaranteed to change things for the better. Your purpose not only changes you for the better, it also changes those around you.

Personal Growth means you are doing the work to grow towards becoming the highest version of yourself. Personal Growth means you believe you are powerful, amazing, and a spiritual being who has the light of God and The Universe within you. When you wake up each morning feeling wonderful about yourself, clear on what your purpose is, and you move through the day with focused direction and an internal joy—then you have grown. Then you will be an infectious ray of light for those whom you come into contact with. Then you will know your purpose.

What would you attempt if you knew you would not fail?

Whatever your mind-set is about yourself and your life- that will dictate how you answer that question. Let's look at two secrets that successful people (in life) share before you answer the question:

1. Successful people know that true failure comes only when they give up and quit. So that's not an option- they keep going, so there's no way to fail. If they miss their target, they simply turn a 'bad day into good data', learn from what happened, recalibrate and keep going. We can learn a lot about success when we look at how we missed our target. It teaches us how not do things on our next attempt. You have the ability to set your life up so that you can't fail if you follow this line of thinking.

2. Successful people are addicted to learning and growing. Most successful people 'fail' more times than the average person even attempts at trying new things. Thomas Edison made thousands of unsuccessful attempts at inventing the light bulb and when asked, "Isn't it a shame that with the tremendous amount of work you have done you haven't been able to get any results?" Edison replied with a smile, "Results! Why, man, I have gotten lots of results! I know several thousand things that won't work!"

This line of thinking and creating success in life is attainable for you. But we must ask you a question: Are you coachable? This question can be answered in many different ways, so we want to clarify what we mean here. Are you open-minded? Are you open to growing and learning? Are you teachable? Can you learn new things, or are you closed off to ideas that are different from your current beliefs? This chapter is about your mindset, and 'shifting' your mind to a new place that will serve you, your health and your life. You have a choice with this chapter. You can choose for it to determine your future potential for growth or you can cause it to cut you off from any possibilities which will cause you to remain stuck where you are. We do realize that many of you who are reading this are very happy and don't feel 'stuck' in your life, but regardless, we believe that you are still meant to evolve and grow throughout this gift called 'life.'

> *"Most people let the outside world determine their focus.*
> *Your work is to be a master of your internal thoughts so*
> *that you can control how to respond to the outside world.*
> *Then and only then can you truly create your life!"*

> ~ *Judy Pearson Kobsar*

"When You Change the Way You Look at Things, The Things You Look at Change."

> ~ *Dr. Wayne Dyer*

You can look at a landscape in the beginning of summer and see all the brown and dying grass, or you can look at that same landscape and see the wisps of green that are still present and showing the beauty that it held during spring. What do you choose to focus on? The brown dying grass, or the green that still lives and holds so much life. This is your Mindset in a nutshell. You get to make the rules in your life so why not set yourself up to succeed? It comes down to how you interpret every situation in your life. Your decisions are based on your filters you look through, and those filters are always changing throughout your life. Every new experience that you have, every book you read, each new person you meet or new subject you study will change your lenses and the way that you look at life.

Some of you might be thinking: 'Hey, you don't know my life, it's really hard right now.' Of course, we don't know what is going on personally with you, but we all have a choice of how we respond to life situations that create the path to the life we choose. If you can get this principle, that will be a great gift you have given to yourself and the world will be better for it.

The Three Controlling Forces Of Your Life Energy

Energy is your life force. Remember when you were a kid and you would run everywhere? And you would splash through puddles and you felt so full of life? It all comes down to ENERGY and at the end of the day energy boils down to 2 sources- and they are black and white, there is no gray area here. These two sources are either productive or destructive, a positive or a negative in your life:

1. Your Thoughts - If your thoughts are not positive, then they are destructive and steal from your life energy.
2. Your Food. - If your food is not nutritious then it creates toxicity which lowers your life force.
3. Your Actions - Body movement creates kinetic energy. If you don't move, vitality is weakened.

That's it, it's that simple. Read it again.

Negative thoughts and emotions are a major cause of inflammation in the body. For some people, inflammatory thoughts occur 24 hours/day, 7 days/week causing prolonged activation of your body systems with detrimental consequences. Virtually every chronic mental illness; depression, anxiety, Alzheimer's, Parkinson's are caused by inflammation. To really understand nerve dysfunction and behavior disorders we must consider how inflammation disturbs neurotransmitter activity and brain degeneration from negative emotional stress. Chronic inflammation affects Dopamine, Adrenaline, Melatonin (sleep) and Serotonin (happy) activity. Atrophy (or catabolism) causes an increase in two enzymes; Indoleamine 2 3-dioxygenase and Tryptophan dioxygenase. This causes a re-prioritization of Tryptophan metabolism to produce less serotonin (happy) and melatonin (sleep) so that tryptophan can make more inflammatory chemicals. We can test for neurotransmitter imbalance and then work to restore balance, but we also must address our thought behaviors to affect real, lasting changes.

How You Think is Physically Manifested in Your Cells

As Dr. Candace Pert, Professor, Department of Physiology & Biophysics, Georgetown University School of Medicine explained in her book, Molecules of Emotion- neurotransmitters called peptides carry emotional messages. "As our feelings change, this mixture of peptides travels throughout your body and your brain. And they're 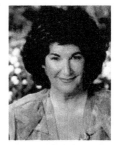 literally changing the chemistry of every cell in your body." So, in fact, 'I think therefore I am' is a very literal experience.

"Thoughts form → Neuropeptides which form → peptides which form → proteins which form → **Physical Structure**

Peptides are the musical notes that allow the orchestra (your body) to play as an integrated symphony. And the music that results is the feeling that you experience as emotions.

Candace Pert PhD; Chief of Brain Biochemistry,
National Institute of Health

The Physics Of Emotion: Don't Believe Everything You Think

Western medicine taught for hundreds of years that your thoughts and emotions are products of your brain and have little to do with your body or your health. We've heard from our wellness partners many times that a practitioner told them, "It's all in your head", thus suggesting that the patients complaint is not real. Pert would say it's all in your "body mind." Emotions are not simply chemicals in your brain: they are electrochemical signals that affect the chemistry and electricity of every cell in your body. The body's electrical state is modulated by emotions so emotional states affect the world outside the body as well. Pert explains, "We're not just little hunks of meat. We're vibrating like a tuning fork- we send out a vibration to other people. You broadcast and receive, you have receptors on every cell in your body that are mini electrical pumps and when activated by a matching 'molecule of emotion' the receptor passes a charge into the cell changing the cell's electrical frequency and its chemistry. Electrochemical messages are passed between brain cells and passed to every cell in your body. Each cell has "receptors," like a "mail box" for electrochemical messages." This is stunning! It means your thoughts are alive and they affect not only you, your body, your decisions, your life . . . but they affect those around you!

How You Think Releases Chemicals That Dictate How You Feel

"Your brain receives information from the world around you and depending on how you interpret this information, your feelings will convert the information into peptides that let you know if there's trouble or cause for celebration. This changes the chemistry of every cell in your body, delivering the energetic effect of whatever your brain is thinking and feeling."

~ *Deepak Chopra MD*

Before Dr. Candice Pert passed away in 2013, she demonstrated that just as your individual cells carry an electrical charge, so does your body. Like an electromagnet generating a field, Pert said that people have a positive charge above their heads and a negative charge below that send 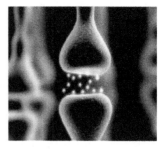 out electrical signals and vibrations. "We're all familiar with one kind of vibration: It's a basic law of physics that when we talk, we send a vibration through the air that someone else perceives as sound but, there are other types of vibrations," Pert explained.

Your Thoughts Program Your Cells

There are thousands of receptors on each cell in your body. Each receptor is specific to one peptide, or protein. When you have feelings of anger, happiness, sadness, if you are excited, or nervous each emotion releases a flurry of neuropeptides which surge through the body and connect with those receptors and change the structure of cells. When one of your cells has been over-exposed to certain peptides due to the negative emotions you are feeling, when that cell divides to become a new cell, it will have more receptors to match the negative peptides compared to the mother cell from which it came. So, if you are bombarding your cells with peptides from negative thoughts, you are programming your cells, and all the new cells to receive more negative peptides in the future. What's even worse is that you're lessening the number of receptors of positive peptides on the cells, making yourself more inclined towards negativity. Go back and read this paragraph again, and then read if 5 more times. We want you to understand the science behind your thoughts so that you have a solid foundation for shifting your mind to change your body and your life.

Here is a table to show you what your body produces when you think and feel a certain way:

Emotion	Body Produces
Exhilarated	Interleukins & Interferon
Tranquility	Valium
Bliss	Endorphins
Acute Stress	Adrenaline/Epinephrine
Chronic Stress	Cortisol
Happy	Serotonin

Here's a deeper understanding into the connection between what your body produces and how medicine works.

This will help you understand the natural power you have within you: Bruce Lipton, PhD stated that "the only reason drugs can have an effect on you is because **your body already makes a natural equivalent to it**. The drugs only can affect you if your cells have a receptor site for the drug and they don't build a receptor site unless your body already makes it. So that means YOU are the creator of your internal world within your body and you are the creator of the external world you experience around you. Yes, things are going to 'happen' to you. But life is just 10% what 'happens' to you and 90% how you respond to it. This is where you begin to understand the power you have to create your life. It begins in your mind.

What Do You Want To Create In Your Life Today?

Become aware of the fact that your energy is responsible for what you attract into your life. This may be a new thought for you, or you may be saying, "Yes! I have seen how it has worked in my life!"

Few are aware of what they attract into their life so we want you to understand that you have more control over your life than you may realize. It's been observed and studied that you will be most like the 5 people you are around most frequently because their energy affects your energy and like attracts like in this universe. So it only makes sense to surround yourself with those who inspire you, lift you up and want you to be and do more with your life! When you do that, you will begin to notice things coming into your life that support your growth. The typical way most people move through life is to make decisions about what is 'good' and what is 'bad' and then go forward chasing the good and pushing away the bad, but meanwhile complaining about the bad, delving into the bad and talking a lot about it. But if you really want to move things quickly and, in your favor, focus all your energy, thoughts and actions on the good. From here you are aligning your energy with what you desire. What you focus on you will get more of. So, if you focus on all the difficulties in your life, you will attract more difficulties in. If you focus on the good in your life or what you WANT to be good in your life, the Universe will provide opportunities for you to have that which you desire.

What Do You Presently Create In Your Personal Life?

To truly RECREATE yourself, you must train and reprogram your mind every day for health just as we are teaching you to train and reprogram your body by the changes you are learning to implement. To be able to handle life without going into overwhelm you must become mentally stronger. You have to develop your brain, so we created the MIND GYM. This is simple process to stimulate stronger nerve pathways in your thoughts that help you avoid mental overload, so you can handle more and bigger challenges in life. As Cesar Torres CEO of the Pivot Point says, *"The thing you should fear most, is being in the same place a year from now as you are today"*.

We all have behaviors or habits that we would like to improve upon. Create a list of 3 that you want to work on. Here are some common examples we have seen over the years:

- Resolve to stop procrastinating with my health.
- Less Judgment. Forgive and accept that we are all on our own path.
- Overcome Fear of _____
- How can I Grow & Learn?
- More Quality time with _____
- Get Organized in my Home Life
- Get Organized in my Professional Life
- No/less Television
- Other _____

MIND GYM

Welcome to Mind Gym. Time to train your brain and build the mental strength to make the most of yourself!

Step 1. Warm Up

Let's start by clearing out mental overload. This is the warm up for your brain. Do you find that you have way too much to do and not enough time to get it done? Do you have a long list of 'to-dos'? What would happen if you lost your To Do list? Would it ruin your day? Would it stress you out? Although a To Do list is wise when you have a lot to do, it is also very taxing on your brain. Your brain only has so much room to store your daily thoughts and things to do. Too much information can cause the brain to freeze up, just like your computer does and you get "BRAIN-LOCK." This is not good if it happens a lot, once in a while is ok, but if it happens all the time, you will soon find that your brain starts missing a beat . . . this is where trouble begins. Mental overload will affect the production of neurotransmitters such a Serotonin and Dopamine. These "calming" brain chemicals get depleted, resulting in emotional upset. Minimize multi-tasking, which is a major source of Cortisol. Many people are "juggling" too many things. Keep your commitments realistic. It may be time to learn to say no to some things and yes to taking care of YOU.

Simple Methods to Break Mental Overload:

- Practice active relaxation. That might be as simple as learning deep breathing, a sauna or steam bath, which elevates body temperature to help discharge stress.
- Prayer or meditation are very powerful and can change your life. Make time to be a human **being**, not a human **doing**. Taking time with family and friends to love and be loved is powerful healing medicine.
- Find your pause button. Discover what that is for you. For us, we enjoy regular exercise, massage, prayer, meditation and runs through the hills. Here is a list of very simple ways to reduce your mental overload and turn some focus towards yourself:

- Call a friend
- Write your feelings in a journal
- Take a 30-minute walk in nature
- Rent an inspirational movie
- Meditate or pray for 15 minutes

- Read a book
- Play with your kids
- Buy or pick some flowers
- Do volunteer work
- Take a yoga class

- Go the gym
- Get a massage
- Take a catnap
- Buy yourself or someone a small present
- Have a heart to heart talk with a friend

- <u>MethodBath</u>: We teach our wellness partners the benefits of baths and many of them love the relaxing 'MethodBath'. Here's the recipe:

  Run a hot bath and pour 2 cups of Epsom salt in, half a cup of baking soda and 10 drops of lavender oil. Soak for 20 minutes to lower your stress, your stress hormones and bring some balance to your systems. We like the Doterra line of essentials oils but there are other options, but be careful to choose the highest quality of oils. Here is a link to our line of oils: **www.doterra.com/US/en/site/wellnessmethod**

- Stick with the things that you can control which is far less than you may imagine. You can't control your kids, your spouse, coworkers, etc. . . . But you can control how YOU respond to them.

Step 2. Lifting Your Life Vision

How much life can you bench press? Does your mental strength allow you to perform the really heavy lifting, so you can create what you want in your life today? When you create a vision for your life you can't start the heavy lifting on the first day but if you start slowly and increase every week you will develop your mental fortitude and build into some serious powerlifting. Life is a gift, we were given this gift for a reason. You need to find your powerful vision for your life and make the most of it. Some of you may feel that focusing on yourself and 'making the most of yourself' is selfish. We are taught to give to others, be charitable and generous. Yes! Keep all those amazing attributes but making the most of yourself is critical and you will inspire others to do more for themselves! When you do this, you will find that you have MORE to give and more to live. THAT will benefit others in the most beautiful way. Vision leads to purpose. When purpose is clear, so are your choices, in fact every choice you make will become aligned with your vision if you can make it clear enough. Vision also creates faith and willpower. Self-doubt is your enemy, so you are really only competing with yourself, while you are striving to attain your own highest standards. Get out of your own way so you can clear your path. To reach your potential is REAL joy and happiness and that can't be bought by any temporary pleasure that wall street is selling. This is what we wish for you in reading this book.

If You Had No Restrictions And Were Guaranteed Success, What Would Your Personal Life Look Like?

Write down your vision quickly, just let it flow. Do not judge what you write or think, get it out of your head and onto paper. Remember, no restrictions—dream fully. Go!

- Spiritual:
- Physical:
- Intellectual:
- Career:
- Primary Relationships: Family
- Secondary Relationships: Friends, coworkers, etc. . . .

Step 3. Core Training

Let's talk about your 'software' which is your brain. In an earlier chapter we shared with you that in one year you will replace 98% of the cells in your body. Everything is replaced except your brain cells and nerve cells- so you can fix your hardware because those cells are in a constant state of recreation, but how do you recreate your software, your core? If nerve cells and brain cells don't replace themselves each year, what can you do to recreate this part of yourself? The good news is that your software can be re-programmed just like a computer. This is how marketing research works to get us to buy their stuff. They sell us happiness, but it's critical to distinguish happiness from pleasure. Slick wall street marketing sells you pleasure in their glossy advertising to convince you that something external can make you happy - but don't be fooled! The junk food, sugary beverages and medications that show an actor on some exotic vacation can give you momentary pleasure- just long enough for you to buy what they are selling. But momentary pleasure and quick fixes will give you a momentary hit of dopamine (the pleasure neurotransmitter in your brain) but it only makes you feel worse in the long run because dopamine blocks serotonin and this will lead to depression. So, in other words, the more pleasure you stimulate in your brain, the more depression will result! We have seen this over and over with our wellness partners who came to work with us. Take control of your life and your health by re-programming your software, training your very core! True happiness comes from within. Dr. Wayne Dyer said, "There is no way to happiness, happiness is the way."

So just do to yourself what society does to you. Market to yourself! The difference is you get to be the programmer of your brain not Wall Street. Use these two elements to program a new behavior: Motivation and Triggers.

1. **Motivation**: 4 Core Motivators:

   • Pleasure and Pain
   • Hope and Fear

As humans we are motivated by moving away from painful experiences in our life. Experiences we no longer want to have. We are motivated by moving towards pleasurable experiences we want to create.

Hope lifts us up to know there is a better future ahead and fear means "False Evidence Appearing Real". So look fear in the eye, face it and move through it.

2. **Triggers/Cues:** Triggers are something in your daily routine that calls you to action. The key to a new behavior is to insert it AFTER something you already do. Here are some examples:

MORNING RITUAL EXAMPLE

Existing Behavior		New Behavior	
After I	Get out of bed	I will	Thank God for the day
After I	Brush my teeth	I will	Drink two glasses of water
After I	Have coffee	I will	Take my vitamins
After I	Get in the car	I will	Ask what I can do to make it a great day

EVENING RITUAL EXAMPLE

Existing Behavior		New Behavior	
After I	Come home	I will	Kiss and hug my wife
After I	Change out of work clothes	I will	Go for a walk and think of one amazing thing that happened today
After I	Put kids to bed	I will	Tell them good night, kiss and hug and say I love you
After I	Get undressed	I will	Write in my journal what I learned today to make tomorrow better

How To Reprogram Your Nervous System

The average person has 60,000 thoughts /day.
95% of them are the SAME thoughts as the day before.

Your nervous system is directly related to your daily thoughts. Thoughts send chemicals to your brain which in turn sends signals to various parts of your body through the spinal cord. How do you advance your thoughts to create the life you desire? Here are 5 steps to progressing your thoughts so that you do not remain stuck playing the same old record in your head:

- **Decide:** Decide what you really want in your life and what is preventing you from having it now.
- **Get Leverage:** Use your motivators of moving away from pain and moving towards pleasure to leverage change.
- **Pattern Interrupt:** Replace negative self-talk with positive talk the same way you learn a new sport. Consistent practice using repetitions.
- **Create:** new experiences and better choices in your life.
- **Condition:** Build mental strength like you do physical strength. Consistent effort over time at the Mind Gym doing mental repetitions. You can't change your muscles after only a week in the gym, your brain works the same way.

Two Forces That Control Your Nervous System— Pain And Pleasure

We are motivated by either moving away from pain or moving towards Pleasure. Pain that exists in our life, whether it be physical pain or emotional pain, is a powerful motivator. Future pain which could become a reality can also motivate us. We are at the same time motivated by an idea, vision or goal that when realized will bring us pleasure.

1. Pain

Change can be painful, we understand this. We've experienced much change in our lives. When we changed our business model many years ago from an insurance-based chiropractic rehabilitation and pain care center to a fully Functional Medicine practice, this was a painful transition for us and it required a lot visits to the Mind Gym. We were in the insurance-based model for years, but when insurance became very limited to the detriment of our patients, we could no longer work in a broken system because too many people needed our help. It all came to a head when we attended a lecture by Dr. Deepak Chopra in Berkeley California.

We asked him how a health care provider can **truly** help patients in the current system? His answer was the catalyst to the massive change that was to come in our lives. He answered, "You can't. The system is set up for profit, not helping patients- so if you truly want to help, you have to leave the system". Stone cold silence fell on the room. Our hearts skipped a beat. He could see our dismay but then he also witnessed our awakening, as did the entire room. We knew he was right but sometimes you have to hear someone else say it. So that's what we did, and it was not easy. Our thoughts were ingrained in the old system and so we had to learn to be entrepreneurs which allowed us to realize our mission, but it was hard, very hard-so we know struggle. We often continue patterns we know are harmful just because it is comfortable much like staying in an unhealthy relationship. But you are designed to grow and evolve, you just need a little push to get started!

Change requires us to do something different which requires effort and it helps to think about who depends on you. Change will bring new thoughts and behavior which will positively affect your relationships because sometimes it's not just about us. Your children, grandchildren, your spouse and family look to you for support throughout their lives. How will it feel if you have to look at them and say "I'm sorry I did not take care of these health issues because it was just too hard to shift my mind to a new way of thinking. I wanted to be there for you, but it was so hard to change." And what about your parents if they are still alive? They gave all they could when you were growing up and now you get the opportunity to give back to them in their time of need. Are you going to be there for them? We know these are hard questions to ask yourself, but pain does control our nervous system and we can use it to our advantage to launch us into changing our thoughts and behaviors. Take your time with this shift, be kind to yourself, but be relentless with your thoughts. You can do it!

2. Pleasure

Instead of thinking about all the things you will have to do, change your focus to all that you will gain when you have made the changes needed. How would that positively affect you in all areas of your life? We are all here to serve a purpose. What greater good are you going to contribute in your community? What legacy will you leave behind? If you are already living your purpose, that is awesome! Let's make sure you can keep doing that. You can't contribute to others if you are struggling with your health. If you have not followed through on making changes in your life it is because you associate too much pain to making those needed changes.

Close your eyes for a moment and imagine who you will be a year from now when you have made the necessary changes in your mind and in your body. Who will that new version of you be? What will you be doing? How will you be spending your days? Get a clear picture of this and feel the pleasure of this vision. That pleasure has the profound power to motivate you to start your process of changing your mind. Let's start your plan to change.

3 LEVELS OF LIFE PLANNING

"Most folks are about as happy as they want to be."

~ Abraham Lincoln

Where Do You Fit Into Your Schedule?

What have you done for yourself today, yesterday, last week? If you don't take care of #1 (YOU), who will? This is an overlooked area of "healing" that is too often put on the back burner. It keeps getting put off until a crisis appears—and then usually it becomes someone else's burden to take care of you (hospital, doctors, care givers, loved ones). Hear us on this- there will NEVER be a 'good' time to start taking care of yourself. Our lives are more full today than the days of our parents and grandparents. You must choose to insert self-care practices into your life. Those of you that aren't busy, you will fill your time up with other things you feel are more important than taking care of yourself. You have to make the time to heal your body. What good are you to your loved ones, co-workers, community groups, if you can't help yourself first? And we've said this before- It is not selfish to focus on yourself. You will be better for those around you, those you care for if you can create the time to focus on yourself.

There are at least 3 stages of the year that you can strategize in order to create the life that you want for yourself and your family rather than just living a pedestrian life. These 3 Stages are:

1. **Daily Crush**
    The small everyday actions and rituals that are the foundation for creating the life you want for yourself.

2. **Weekly Warrior:**

A weekly look ahead to anticipate challenges that will come your way. Set expectations that create a strategy for what you want to create and put in place the everyday practice that leads you to the outcomes you want for your life. We call the weekly strategy your SPARK for the week which is an acronym for the different areas of your life:

- **SPARK**

    S piritual: 5 Day Mental Cleanse to start removing negative thought patterns.

    P hysical: Exercise and Diet plan for the week

    A dventures: Have Fun! Plan things to do just for fun, life is short

    R elationships: Connect to people! Family, friends and neighbors.

    K now your financial score. More stress is created in life from this one area.

3. **Magical Mastery:**

As the daily crush turns into weekly warriors, we move into quarters (micro cycles) and years (macrocycles):

- **Microcycle**   A 7-week plan for each quarter of the year ahead
- **Macrocycle**   A one-year plan that anticipates a lot of growth in your career when work is busy and when work is slower, you can plan for personal growth.

Life is a result of an accumulation of days, weeks, months and years. These cycles all come together and define who we become as people and the life we create. There will be times that you fall off the track but if you stay the course, you get to join the few that we call the **Masters.** Let's dive deeper into each of these and go into more detail:

1. Daily Crush

By living each day with purpose, we can create a Magical Life. 'Make' the life you dream about, don't just leave it to chance. All you have to do is schedule yourself to create the daily magic based on your goals in a Daily Crush Journal.

Start with a morning power question (AM PQ). i. e. : What is going to be great about today? What am I grateful for today?
Set the tone for your day with an empowered state of mind. Think of your mind, your emotions and your spirit as the ultimate garden. The way to ensure a bountiful, nourishing harvest is to plant seeds like love, warmth and appreciation — instead of seeds of disappointment, anger and fear. Use them to bring fulfillment and abundance to your life, and as an antidote to negative emotions.

4 Power Emotions

Life is a GIFT. We live everyday with that in our hearts and use a daily reminder of the acronym **GIFT:**

- **G**ratitude the single greatest power to change your life by instantly changing a negative state to positive.
- Intention/purpose: How can you become great? Every great leader finds their purpose to create valuable change in the world. When you live your purpose, nothing is a boring

or a chore. Those who learn the power of contribution experience deep joy and true fulfillment because you serve something larger than yourself and life takes on a deeper meaning. There's no richer emotion than the sense that who you are as a person, adds to the life of someone you care about deeply or even a total stranger.

- Faith: When you experience the power of unshakable faith, you have all the confidence you need. Love is the most powerful force in the universe. It can overcome anything.
- Total Passion: is the force that awakens you. Passion blows the lid off of your limitations. It shakes your mind free and breaks your old patterns of thinking.

The Power of Questions

The quality of your life improves with the quality of your questions. Asking yourself questions is one of the simplest and most powerful tools to change your thoughts.

Questions that Empower You	Questions that Disable you
• What can I learn from this? • What's great about this situation? • What results do I want to produce? • What am I willing to do to make this the way I want it? • What must I stop doing in order to make this the way I want it? • How can I do this and enjoy the process? • What do I really want?	• Why does this always happen to me? • Why me? • Why can't I do anything right? • Why can't I make this work? • What did I do wrong? • What's wrong with me?

How To Apply Empowering Questions

1. Think of a challenging situation that you currently have and write it down.
2. What are the dis-empowering questions you've been asking yourself regarding this situation?
3. What are some empowering questions you can ask yourself to move towards a positive resolution? Here's some examples:

- What's great about this?
- What's not perfect yet?
- What am I willing to do to make things the way I want it?
- What am I willing to no longer do?
- How can I do what's necessary and enjoy the process?

Weekly Warrior

As days become weeks, life will present challenges that distract us from our purpose. Sometimes life can hit pretty hard, but we can keep going forward if we have a Warrior's mentality. Anticipate the problems, you will encounter on the life path and plan how you will deal with them. Try to make this fun! Winning in life is done by taking the hits and still moving forward. Set personal development goals for each week. At the end of the weeks, look back and evaluate how you did. As you move through this you will become a **Weekly Warrior.**

Micro Cycles: 7 Weeks

Choose an area of your life where you want to grow and focus on it for one micro cycle (7 weeks). It can be spiritual, financial, emotional, relationships, etc. Here is an example of physical goals. You would typically choose one but if they complement each other you can choose more.

Physical Workout Type: Weeks: ____	☐ **Strength**
	☐ **Weight Loss**
	☐ **Flexibility**
	☐ **Metabolic Rehabilitation /Energy**
	☐ **Anti-aging**
	☐ **Stability/Balance**
	☐ **Structural Balance (Posture)**
	☐ **Condition Specific:**
	Diabetes / Hormones / Thyroid / Insomnia / Pain/ Digestion/ other: _____
	£ Sport Specific:
	Triathlete/ Dance / Tennis / Swim/ Other: _____

Mastery Macrocycles: 1 Year

A master is rarely in reaction to life because they are creating the life they want for themselves, so they always anticipate what is coming and they already have a plan in place. A true master looks at the year in advance and anticipates the seasons throughout the year. Here are some important questions to ask yourself to set yourself up to succeed at becoming a master of your destiny.

1. When is your personal life most busy?
2. When is it most slow?
3. When is your work life most busy?
4. When is it most slow?
5. When do you typically get sick?
6. When are you most energetic and vital?

Answering these questions allows you to know how much time and energy you have available at different times of the year, so you can decide the following in advance:

1. When to push harder and when to back off.
2. How to budget your finances so you know when to expect more money coming in and when to be more conservative.
3. When to go on holidays and spend more family time.
4. When to focus on building your financial wealth.
5. When to be extra careful with your health and conserve your energy.

You have now learned about the Mind Gym, so now it is time to experience it! Follow these exercises to start training your brain for success. You will begin to notice little things changing at first, and then will witness an unfolding of opportunities and experiences that you never thought possible.

Here's some action steps to help you change your thoughts and change your habits. We want to show you that change doesn't mean you have to be deprived of your old habits. It means you will be replacing that habit with a new one that will serve you. Come up with some new behaviors to begin reprogramming your mind and thoughts.

ACTION STEPS

What do I need or want more of?

Choose one area of your life that you checked off from the 'Lifting Your VISION' section and pick one specific thing that you can do to improve it.

- Spiritual: Purpose, Meaning
- Physical Health:
- Intellectual:
- Career:
- Connection and community
    - Primary Relationships: Family
    - Secondary Relationships: Friends, coworkers, etc. . . .

1. **Motivation**: 4 Core Motivators
    - Pleasure and Pain.
        - What is the pain and discomfort you have with making changes?
        - What pleasure would you get from making changes in your life right now?
    - Hope and Fear
        - What are the costs of not changing?
        - What will you gain from changing?

2. **Triggers/Cues:** Come up with some new behaviors to begin reprogramming your mind and thoughts. Use the example below to guide you.

MORNING RITUAL EXAMPLE

Existing Behavior		New Behavior	
After I	Get out of bed	I will	Thank God for the day

EVENING RITUAL EXAMPLE

Existing Behavior		New Behavior	
After I	Come home	I will	Kiss and hug my wife

Understand and Influence Your Behavior

Identify your crucial moments. Identify the time, place, and/or people that most tempt you to fall back. Some examples:	Create vital behaviors. What can you do when you are at risk? Refocus your mind or change your state so you don't succumb to the urge, for just 3 or 4 minutes.
After 7: 30 pm at night, tired and defenses are weak	Get out of the house and go for a 20-minute walk
When "the game is on" it triggers pizza and hot dogs.	Watch the game at the gym on the treadmill or stationary bike.
Movie theaters trigger popcorn.	Bring a healthy snack with you
TV commercials at home on the couch trigger snacking	- 10 jumping jacks/ 10 push ups - play with your kids or your pet

WHO AM I

I am your greatest helper or heaviest burden.
I will push you onward or drag you down to failure.
I am completely at your command.
Half the things you do you might just as well turn over to me, and I will be able to do them quickly, correctly.
I am easily managed - you must merely be firm with me. Show me exactly how you want something done, and after a few lessons I will do it automatically.
I am the servant of all great people; and alas, of all failures as well. Those who are failures, I have made failures.
I am not a machine, though I work with all the precision of a machine plus the intelligence of a human being.
You may run me for a profit or turn me for ruin - it makes no difference to me.
Take me, train me, be firm with me, and I will place the world at your feet.
Be easy with me and I will destroy you.
Who am I
I AM YOUR HABIT.

Anonymous

REDUCING INFLAMMATION

The Silent Killer

*Inflammation underlies up to 98%
of the diseases afflicting humans.*

~ Annals of the New York Academy of Science, 2005.

Inflammation is the underlying cause of heart disease, cancer, diabetes, Alzheimer's, Parkinson's, obesity, . . . we could go on and on, but you get the picture. It even causes joint and muscle pain, which is often given the worthless label discussed earlier called 'arthritis'. In fact, you can attach the Greek term "itis" to any body part, and that means it is inflamed. So, neuritis simply means nerve inflammation, tendonitis is tendon inflammation, gastritis; stomach inflammation, hepatitis; liver inflammation, myocarditis; heart inflammation, arthritis simply means joint inflammation, and so on.

How Inflammation Affects Every Aspect Of Your Body

The fact is, if any body part or organ is inflamed, its ability to function is compromised. Every organ in your body can be affected by inflammation.

- Heart Inflammation => Shortness of breath, fluid retention, heart failure.
- Stomach Inflammation => Irritable Bowel disease, crohns, malnutrition.
- Liver Inflammation => high blood pressure, cholesterol, blood sugar.
- Lung Inflammation => COPD; asthma, bronchitis, emphysema

Every day as we review the labs test results, we see that 90 percent of people have stomach or 'gut inflammation' from the toxins in food and beverages consumed. If your stomach is inflamed, you can't digest your food which means you can't get the nutrients to your cells. You can eat the best organic food from the farmers market but, if you can't assimilate the nutrients, they are just passing through and your health will suffer. Similarly, if you can't digest the vitamin supplements you are taking because your stomach is inflamed, you won't realize the benefits from them. Here are some common symptoms of gut inflammation:

- **Restless Sleep** leaves you confused, irritable, moody.
- **Muscle tone** is fading, and it feels like parts of your body are just withering away.
- **Fatigue.** That energy you used to enjoy is a shadow of its former self.
- **Stubborn fat** on your belly, hips, thighs, and chest area starting to feel permanent.

- **Digestive distress and constipation** . . . but you're told it's all just a normal part of growing old.
- **Sore muscles, swollen joints**. Forget about playing with the kiddos! You're told you are past your prime.

The first step to restoring your health is often to reduce inflammation. Inflammation is a beneficial process when white blood cells and chemicals protect us from bacteria and viruses. However, when your immune system mistakenly triggers an inflammatory response when no threat is present, chronic low-grade inflammation occurs causing autoimmune disease, fibromyalgia, cancer, etc.

How Does Inflammation Begin?

Every single day we breathe in chemicals from the air and consume them in water we drink. Our water is full of chemicals that are put there to 'clean' it. These chemicals are hormone disruptors. We eat and drink processed products that alter our digestive and detoxification capacities. Our body has normal detoxification processes that are naturally detoxing 24 hours a day. The liver is our main detoxification organ, but we also detoxify through our kidneys, bowels, sweat glands, and respiratory system. Our daily choices often hinder the function of our detoxification systems, which adversely affects our bodily functions. Our daily choices are causing the systems of our body to become inflamed. We want you to know the 3 main drivers of inflammation, and then we'll give you some steps to reduce it:

1. Physical Trauma
2. Chemical Toxins
3. Emotional Stress

Inflammation Is A Fire Inside Every Fat Cell Of Your Body.

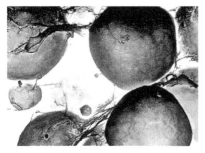 The fire that may be burning in your body is fueled by toxic molecules, and those toxins char your body from the inside-out. Medical experts everywhere agree: Inflammation is at the root of 98% of heart disease, cancer, diabetes, and hundreds of other conditions are accelerated when these inflammatory molecules are released. The result? Your metabolism shuts down, and your body is forced to eat away at your organs and muscles in order to survive. And here is what's even worse . . . fat cells leak out toxins that age and inflame your body. So, the last thing you want is a billion leaky fat cells that are toxic sewage dumps waiting to deposit inside your body. But with a sedentary lifestyle, poor food choices, poisons in the air and water . . . as you approach the age of 35, your fat cells begin to 'leak', it's inevitable.

Are YOUR Fat Cells Leaking? Instead of releasing healthy fatty acids for your metabolism to burn as energy, they spew out deadly inflammatory molecules such as IL-1 (Interleukin 1) and TNFa (Tumor Necrosis Factor alpha). These 'septic' molecules are like acid in your system, that dissolves living tissue over time and rapidly age you. You start to feel symptoms of aging when this is happening, yet many have trouble expressing what exactly is going on . . . something just doesn't feel right. Leaky fat cells also create a condition known as "Fatty Liver". This means your liver can no longer process sugars or carbohydrates. So, you get fat. And you get sick. And your risk for diseases such as Diabetes, Alzheimer's, Heart Disease and Cancer skyrocket.

Why Inflammation Must Be Addressed At Its Root

The fact that your immune system drives the inflammatory process in disease is well established. Unfortunately, conventional healthcare offers little in the way of solutions to overcoming the chronic inflammatory diseases. The conventional approach is to suppress inflammation with medications which does not stop the underlying disease processes or allow for damaged tissues to heal. Imagine your body is your house, and your house is on fire and all you did is suppress the flames but still allow the coals to burn causing more damage until eventually your entire house (body) is destroyed. Unless you switch off the cause of the fire (inflammation), all you have done is masked the symptoms and allowed the disease process to continue destruction of your cells, tissues and organs. Every day we see commercials on TV for medications designed to mask pain and inflammation. The Opiod problem in our country has been allowed to skyrocket over the past 10 years and it is an incredibly sad situation. No amount of drugs will resolve the underlying problem and yet the images on the screen tell you that the drug will restore your health and you'll do a happy dance on a beach in Fiji.

Acute and Chronic Inflammation

Why does some inflammation get better after a short time, while other times it goes on and on and on . . . seemingly forever (in some sad cases it is forever!) The reason is there are two different kinds of inflammation that you can experience:

1. Acute Inflammation: A single trauma causes damage and the immune system is alerted to repair and remove damaged cells. Damaged, dead cells initiate peripheral inflammation, which is perpetuated by "living" cells that arrive to heal and release more inflammatory chemicals. This explains acute inflammation.

2. <u>Chronic Inflammation:</u> Repeated trauma (chemicals, emotions or physical force) occurs over an extended period which creates an imbalance of systems of the body—immune, structural, hormone, etc. Low symptoms of sickness begin to appear which eventually become a disease caused by system dysregulation: i. e. ; diabetes, depression, irritable bowels, sleep, chronic pain, etc. All of them come with a boat load of symptoms associated with complex inflammation that can only be addressed by therapies that target the systems of your body on a global level. Chronic inflammation is at the heart of weight gain, accelerated aging and virtually every disease and it is why we see the following:

- Heart Attack: 100% Increased Risk
- Type 2 Diabetes: 160% Increased Risk
- Skin Cancer: 70% Increased Risk

The Truth About Detoxification For Reducing Inflammation

Detoxification programs have become a huge business, yet we also regularly hear doctors claim such programs are nonsense or that our bodies already have the ability to detoxify. This is true, but you must support your detox pathways to ensure proper cellular metabolism, neutralize metabolic by-products and removing toxins. What we will be sharing with you is the science of how your body gets rid of waste. If waste builds up in your body, you get sick and fat. That's not 'our opinion', that is the science of how the body works. So, the key to reducing the toxins in your body is to learn how to first; enhance your body's capacity to detoxify and get rid of waste on its own, and second; how to minimize your exposure to toxins.

How To Know If You Are Toxic?

TEST! Don't guess. We have a short quiz you can take on our website and if it suggests you are toxic, the next step is a blood test to assess the severity of your toxic load that is creating inflammation. Here are some tests for chronic inflammation:

- *Homocysteine:* a blood test for methylation mutations. This means less Phase 2 detoxification enzymes leading to atrophy.
- *C- reactive protein:* a blood test to measure a protein that signals inflammation.
- *C-reactive cardiac protein:* a blood test that is the best predictor of stroke and heart attack.
- *ESR (sed rate) test:* a blood test for non-specific indicators of inflammation.
- *Organic acid test:* urine test to measure sulfur which is peed out when inflammation causes atrophy from the loss of mitochondria mostly found in muscle.

Inflammation And Accelerated Aging

Briana was only 49. Some people age prematurely, do you feel like this?

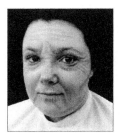

Do you feel like you are aging prematurely? Much like an autoimmune disease like ALS, Lupus, Psoriasis, or Thyroid Dysfunction, these inflammatory molecules force your body to turn against itself. Then what you have are thousands of these molecules all working like an army of the walking dead, running rampant inside your aging body. Have you ever seen someone who looked 10 or even 20 years older than their actual age? Maybe when you look in the mirror that's how you feel when you see your image staring back at you. So, if you look older than you should, then your body may be producing molecules that steal your health and ravage your body by destructive inflammation. When we are toxic, the mechanism for detoxification gets sluggish, and toxins stay active longer. If you have experienced the frustration of trying to lose weight, doing everything right with diet and exercise, but the weight just won't come off, it is often because the toxins trigger fat storing.

When your body is healthy, the process of detoxification runs effortlessly but when the detoxification mechanism in your liver gets sluggish, toxins get backed up into your bloodstream and pollute your body and you get sick. If you are overweight, you are often toxic because pesticides, heavy metals, plastics are stored in fat cells and as you empty your fat cells, you need to flush out the toxins that are dumped into your blood and poison your metabolism which impairs weight loss. Excess weight and obesity aside, nearly every disease on the planet has links to toxicity.

Toxic Load There is no question that you are toxic- everyone is. The question is "how toxic are you?" To answer this, you must understand the 'toxic load'. Think of total toxic load like a glass filling over with water. It takes a certain amount to fill the glass and at a certain point it spills over. When our detoxification system is overloaded, we get symptoms of sickness, but it may take years of accumulated toxic stress to get to that point. The role of toxins and detoxification in health has been largely ignored by medicine because most doctors utilize pharmaceuticals in lieu of getting to the root cause, which actually contributes to the toxic load. Thankfully, scientists and some practitioners are starting to recognize its importance in health. Many of you may have symptoms of toxicity that you don't recognize. Our quiz reveals your toxic load- you can take it here: <u>found on our website member section www.mywellnessmethod.com</u>. Detoxifying might be the critical missing piece for you to reclaim your health and feel good again.

Inflammation And Autoimmune Disease

You may have heard the term 'Autoimmune Disease'—but what exactly does it mean? An autoimmune condition is when your body's immune system becomes hyper-active due to inflammatory stress and begins an attack on your own body tissues and organs. Inflammation triggers an autoimmune response in your body from poor diet, infections, medications, hormones among others. The autoimmune response breaks down your intestinal/gut lining causing it to become porous like a sponge. When your intestinal lining becomes porous it allows partially undigested food, toxins, viruses, yeast, and bacteria to pass through into your bloodstream. This is known as leaky gut syndrome (LGS). The truth of the situation is that FOOD MATTERS. That's right, it's not just a movie (which by the way you should watch), it's a major trigger to kick off autoimmune issues.

When the intestinal lining is repeatedly damaged, the gut is unable to use the nutrients and enzymes that are vital to proper digestion. It may sound relatively harmless, but this situation leads to a loss of nutrients which affects our health and we respond with mild symptoms that end up in serious and debilitating disease. Since your immune system can become overburdened, these inflammatory triggers are cycled continuously through your blood where they affect cells, tissues and organs. You can now begin to see how diseases develops. Waxing and waning of symptoms is par for autoimmunity. When stress is high a person will 'flare up'. Work stress, poor diet, restless sleep will cause intestinal permeability to increase and food will leak through. Now that you know this disease process of your body, the main point we are trying to make here is DON'T WAIT!

Tissues of The Body Affected By Autoimmune Attack

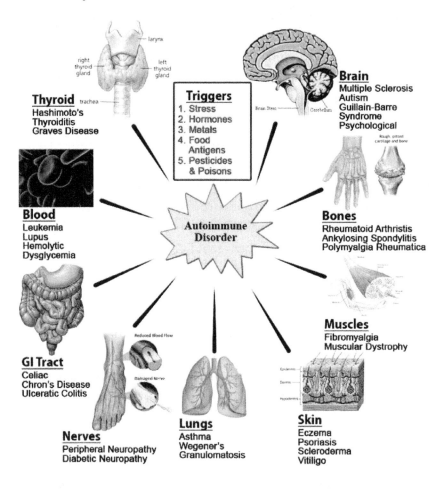

Triggers
1. Stress
2. Hormones
3. Metals
4. Food Antigens
5. Pesticides & Poisons

Thyroid
Hashimoto's
Thyroiditis
Graves Disease

Brain
Multiple Sclerosis
Autism
Guillain-Barre Syndrome
Psychological

Blood
Leukemia
Lupus
Hemolytic
Dysglycemia

Bones
Rheumatoid Arthristis
Ankylosing Spondylitis
Polymyalgia Rheumatica

Autoimmune Disorder

Muscles
Fibromyalgia
Muscular Dystrophy

GI Tract
Celiac
Chron's Disease
Ulceratic Colitis

Nerves
Peripheral Neuropathy
Diabetic Neuropathy

Lungs
Asthma
Wegener's
Granulomatosis

Skin
Eczema
Psoriasis
Scleroderma
Vitiligo

How Inflammation Affects Your Brain

"If inflammatory processes could be identified and harnessed, then brain function may be protected during aging and age related degenerative diseases through preventing inflammation."

~ Dr. Kobsar;
The Journal of Nutritional Perspectives, April 2018

Your brain and nerve tissue are among the first tissues affected by inflammation. This leads to degeneration which affects all mental function including brain fog, memory loss, depression, anxiety, which eventually result in:

- Alzheimer's: 184% Increased Risk
- Dementia: 45% Increased Risk

Depression often results when your body attempts to protect itself from inflammation using hormones and neurotransmitters. Symptoms of depression associated with inflammation include flat mood, slow thinking, isolation, altered perceptions, bipolar disorder and postpartum depression. At the same time, cortisol (stress hormone that buffers inflammation) sensitivity goes down which alters communication in your nervous system by stimulating the Vagus nerve, which connects your gut and brain. Inflammation also causes Tryptophan to steal from the production of serotonin (happy) and melatonin (sleep), which triggers anxiety and irritation.

Action Steps To Detoxification

We work with our wellness partners all over the world to help them reduce inflammation and every one of them is grateful they took that first step and didn't wait any longer. A year from now, you will wish you started today. So, let's get you started!

Depending on your symptoms, genetics and environment, you will need a personalized strategy to eradicate toxins and replenish essential nutrients to detoxify your systems for optimal health. As you work through each step outlined below, think of these as the 'big picture' approach to enhance detoxification. They will begin to help you correct problems caused by toxicity, and help you safely eliminate stored toxins. None of them are quick fixes because there are no quick fixes. Begin with these tips and simple action steps to get you started right away to reduce inflammation and as always, find a reputable functional medicine practitioner to help guide you.

Action Steps

Start with our Detox Quiz found on our website member section www.mywellnessmethod.com to detect any signs of toxicity by ascertaining your level of toxic load and whether a blood test is needed for you to answer the question: What do I need to remove?

- **Infectious** (bacteria, ticks, yeast, parasites, prions)
- **Processed Food**
- **Allergens** (food, mold, dust, animal products, pollens, chemicals)
- **Stress** (physical and/or emotional)

Lab tests determine where inflammation is present in your body. First identify troubled areas through proper lab tests, then start a natural detoxification to address the affected areas using the following steps:

Action Step #1—Toxic Chemical Removal:

We are exposed to 6 million pounds of mercury and 2. 5 billion pounds of chemical toxins every year. The Environmental Working Group reports the average newborn has 287 known toxins in their blood, so imagine how many you have been exposed to in your lifetime?

The truth is we are living in a sea of pollution. Eighty thousand toxic chemicals have been released into our environment since the industrial revolution, and very few have been tested for their long-term health impact. Free radicals in air pollution is up to 300x more damaging that cigarette smoke. How can we not be affected by all these poisons? We either detoxify or we store them. Eliminating as many as you can is critical for healing. You can't totally eliminate all of them, but you can make an impact with a good quality air filter in your bedroom, where you sleep and breathe deeply every night for 8 hours! Go to our website to see our preferred and approved air filter system. A good quality detox once a year is a great solution. There are many to choose from. Our 28 Day Wellness Method Detox is effective and easy- so anyone can do it!

Action Step #2—Heavy Metal Removal:

Mining, burning fossil fuels, use of phosphates for sewage, farming and industrial manufacturing leads to heavy metals. We all have them and they disrupt our repair enzymes. We get aluminum from cookware, baking powder, tap water, processed foods, car exhaust, deodorants, antacids. Wild caught fish have mercury while paint and makeup often contain lead. Heavy metals tangle up the nerves in our brain (neurofibrillary tangles) and make a gluey substance (amyloid) that gum up the brain function. One way to reduce amyloid production is **Phosphatidylserine (PS)** to perk your memory and stave off Alzheimer's.

Action Step #3—Pesticide Reduction:

Pesticides in our water and non-organic produce cause damage. This is reported in Science Daily and Journal of the American Medical Association. A good quality water filter is a great place to start and eating organic produce only. Go to our website to see our preferred and approved air filter system.

Action Step #4—Alcohol and Cigarette Smoke Reduction:

Alcohol is metabolized into acetaldehyde and leads to nervous system damage. Cigarette smoke has 4,800 chemicals and each puff of smoke contains 10 trillion free radicals. Avoid these wherever possible.

Action Step #5—Heal Your Stomach:

Bad Stuff Out. Probiotics can help but until you reduce the inflammation healing cannot start so you must eliminate inflammatory, refined foods (flour and sugar), omega-6 oils like corn, soy and safflower oils. Dairy has over 60 hormones that contribute to imbalances, so removal of dairy is recommended. Cows make hormones that are natural for them, but not natural for us humans, so organic milk does not help with this problem. They are also injected with hormones and anti-biotics.

Good Stuff In. Eat a whole, real, unprocessed, organic diet. Simple steps like choosing organic food and drinking filtered water will minimize anti-biotics, toxins and hormone imbalance. Consider doing our Anti-Inflammatory Detox Diet- you can inquire about that on our website.

Action Step #6—Flushing the Liver:

The liver is a filter that detoxifies your body, protects you from harmful chemicals, elements in food, environmental toxins, and your own waste products of metabolism. Medications, alcohol, plastics, processed food and excess vitamin supplements impair liver function which results in excess estrogen, insulin and cortisol while lowering thyroid hormone and testosterone. Gluten has been shown to damage the liver's capacity to cleanse the blood of estrogen.

Action Step #7—Detox Your Spirit:

This is just as important as detoxing your body. We create toxins just by being overwhelmed, depressed, and stressed. Being alone in nature is a good start. Practicing mindfulness, meditation, prayer, and deep breathing exercises are also great ways to quiet the mind. Listening to music, reading an uplifting book and turning OFF the news can reset your mind and spirit.

Action Step #8—Eliminate daily:

Constipation causes waste toxicity to build up in your intestines and back up in your blood to gum up your precious filters (i. e. ; liver and kidneys). This will lead to back-up into the liver hormones and cause over production of estrogen, insulin and cortisol. You must be able to eliminate the toxic contents within your intestines. We use 'Smooth Moves Tea' or CascaraSagrada with many wellness partners to help 'get them moving' and to increase their water intake.

Progress Is Not Always A Straight Line

Since complex systems change in a non-linear fashion, we expect progress to be up and down. That means getting better can be a matter of two steps forward and one step back which can make it difficult to assess improvement. For this reason, we look at how you are trending so that short setbacks don't sabotage a winning game plan. Keep in mind the idea of trajectory. If you slowly push that ball up a hill for long enough, you may fall a few times, but you eventually get over the hump, and see a big jump in progress. Problems aren't solved by quick fixes like turmeric, goji berries, or anti-inflammatory drugs. They require a strategy to regulate systemic health - diet, exercise, sleep, and stress regulation. These are the fundamentals that get ignored in favor of a magic pill.

ENDOCRINE SYSTEM

Regimen
Educational Curriculum
Coaching
Reducing Inflammation
Endocrine System
Alignment of Your Structure
Total Nutrition
Exercise

Hormones, The Chemical Messengers

To control your hormones is to control your life.

~ Dr. Barry Sears MD

Case Study: A Note From Judy

At 44 years old, I gave birth to our youngest daughter and she was healthy, thriving and a joy. I was the complete opposite. I became lethargic, depressed and a horror to be around. We considered it to be post-natal depression caused by hormone imbalances, and it was causing much distress in our family. I couldn't fully enjoy our new baby and I felt like such a burden on the family and began to lose a sense of myself. It was a push every single day to get up and get moving, I was cold all the time, my body hurt, I was sad, I had a hard time sleeping, my hair was getting thin and I felt an overall sense of doom. It was a very difficult time. As things continued longer than they should have, Dr. Kobsar began his deep dive to finding the underlying cause of this starting with lab tests. About that same time, I was at my OBGYN for a routine post-baby checkup and we discussed my problem and she suggested I get my labs done so she could look at my hormone levels. Easy enough since the lab was right there, so out of curiosity I went to see how her lab findings would compare to Dr. Kobsar's results.

She diagnosed me with an under productive thyroid—commonly known as hypothyroidism which is when your thyroid does not produce enough hormones for what is needed. She prescribed Synthroid which is one of the standard drugs for this condition. Synthroid is a synthetic form of thyroid hormone - thyroxine or T4. Women who are put on Synthroid typically are on it for life. I did not take the medication and waited for Dr. Kobsar's lab tests. The lab 'normals' in the insurance medical system are based on 'average' ranges. The lab ranges we use in functional medicine are based on optimally healthy ranges- more on that later. Dr. Kobsar reviewed my functional medicine labs and found that I had Hashimoto's Thyroiditis—an autoimmune condition that hinders thyroid hormone production but is different from hypothyroidism, and a medication like Synthroid is not going to do anything to help with this issue.

It was such a relief to know what was going on with me! I had begun to think I was never going to feel normal again and that my family relationships were always going to be a struggle. My condition had turned what should have been a joyful time in our lives into one of struggle and depression. Now, with the correct diagnosis- everything made sense and we went to work on resolving the root cause.

Things began to level out within a couple months using The Wellness Method to reduce toxins, alter my diet, reduce stress, custom made whole food supplements, a change to my exercise regimen and some mind set/shift practice. Because of our Wellness Method, I was able to balance my hormones, but if I had not been educated about resolving the root cause of health issues I would be on thyroid medication that do not work and still suffering from the symptoms of Hashimoto's. My function as a mother would suffer, my relationship with my husband would be a disaster, my self-esteem would be low and the inevitable weight gain that goes with this disease would contribute to all above factors. But through our approach, today I am healthier now than I was in my 20's and 30's. I'm thriving, totally clear headed, emotionally balanced and on fire to help others!

Our endocrine system is responsible for so much of our body functions. Those teeny tiny little, microscopic hormones govern our very way of life. They literally have the ability to ruin relationships, end marriages, lose jobs and rob you of your joy. I experienced some of this and we see this every day in our practice. Thankfully we are able to help these issues and get people back to enjoying life again. I am walking talking, living proof that we MUST address the endocrine system and get our hormones back in balance and then keep them there! You can do this, but you have to be willing to invest in yourself— but really, I always say, why wouldn't you do that? It's the best return on investment you can ever make.

Hormones, The Chemical Messengers

Hormones are an enormous and often-overlooked reason for illness and disease. Hormones are the messengers that direct all the chemical reactions (metabolism) in of your body that are essential for life. We would not be able to survive without hormones. Your endocrine system is made up of tissues and glands that secrete hormones into the blood to deliver messages to the cells. We must also include the hormones of the brain and nervous system called neurotransmitters, when discussing the Endocrine System to give a complete picture. Neurotransmitters are not defined as hormones in the classic sense, but they function the same. Hormones are messenger molecules of your endocrine systems while neurotransmitters are messenger molecules of your brain and nervous systems.

There Are No Bad Hormones

Balancing hormones is critical to your health and yet many people are living in disharmony with their natural biorhythms which are controlled by hormones. We depend on them to keep us in a healthy balance, but the fact is they are running haywire in many people. It becomes easy to understand why so many Americans are sick, tired, overweight and depressed when we look at their hormone lab tests in our clinic every day. When you learn how to balance your systems, you will understand the importance of managing these tiny messengers. You might have thought "I'm tired of feeling crappy all the time. Do I need to do hormone replacement or, is there a natural way to feel better?" We have these conversations all the time, and we want to assure you that in most cases you can balance your hormones naturally without medications. All the hormones in your body are necessary and introducing a hormone drug can wreak even more havoc to your hormone balance. So, how do you know if they are in or out of balance?

Test! Don't Guess

The only way to know is to test them. Some are best tested in the blood, some in the saliva, it just depends on which hormone. But testing is just one important step. The second important step is to ask how the tests are interpreted. **In the insurance health system, lab test 'normal ranges' are derived by the average of all the sick people that came before you to the lab.** Yes, you read that right. The "normal" lab values have nothing to do with "healthy normal" standards, they are based on an "average normal" bell curve based on all the tests that lab did from everyone that came to that lab. This makes us crazy! Hear us on this: this means a lab in northern California will have different "normal" reading then a lab in southern California because the ranges are based on the averages of all of those that get their blood drawn at that lab. Do your research and you will be as puzzled and disturbed as we were to discover this fact.

Question: What kind of people are sent for labs?

That's right, for the most part they are sick people. They went to their doctor because they didn't feel good and their doctor sent them for lab tests. Do you really want the average 'normal' from all the sick people to be used as your gold standard? Let that sink in a moment. It's true that some healthy people get labs for a yearly physical, but by far the majority that have lab tests are sick. This is how lab normal ranges are derived, which brings us to the 'prescribed treatment'. The lab results dictate your doctor's decisions to prescribe medications or surgery!

My Labs Are Normal But I Don't Feel Normal

You may not have a 'healthy' liver but you have a 'normal' liver. You aren't **sick enough** to require medication or surgery. Has this ever happened to you? This is the healthcare system saying 'you aren't sick enough to need medications so we will wait until you are.'

If you are experiencing any of the following symptoms, your hormones may be out of balance, so ask yourself if any of these things apply to you:

- Are you overweight and putting on more belly fat?
- Are you depressed?
- How do you sleep . . . are you tired but wired?

- Do you need caffeine to get started in the morning and a glass of wine at night to wind down the day?
- Does your mood and energy level swing up and down?
- Do you crave sugar or salt?
- As a woman, do you have premenstrual syndrome, painful or heavy periods and a low sex drive?

The Endocrine System - A Precise Musical Symphony

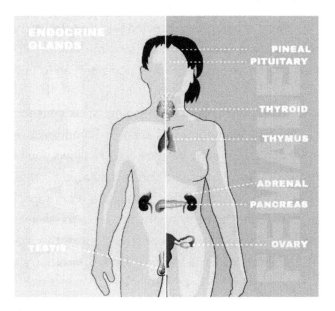

Hormones and neurotransmitters perform together in harmony, like musical instruments in a magnificent symphony to control your metabolism. Problems start when one instrument gets out of tune and the musical conductor (your brain), sends the wrong signals to your body to control everything from stress (via adrenal glands); to blood sugar (via our pancreas); to energy (thyroid); to sex drive (via reproductive organs). Hormones are transported in the blood to the target cells with hormone receptors. Once the hormones reach their target cell, they control your metabolism.

Hormones also control your mood, sleep, growth, repair and more. This requires the harmonious integration of all biological systems that is possible only if all organs, and systems can efficiently communicate. Hormones interpret your environmental stimuli into chemical reactions in your body. The chemical reactions dictate which one of two states your metabolism will conduct itself within. At any given time, your metabolism can be either Catabolic or Anabolic:

1. Catabolic: breaking down fat, protein and carbohydrates. Once these are gone we break down muscles and organs.
2. Anabolic: making enzymes, building muscle, repairing DNA This is where we spend most of our sleeping hours.

Since your environment is always changing, so is your metabolism. Sometimes it's hot, sometimes it's cold. Sometimes we stress, sometimes we don't. Hormone balance is what allows you to adapt to your environment. Hormone secretion is regulated by what is called a "negative feedback system:" that acts like a barn door, i.e., when blood sugar gets high, the body opens the door to let insulin out to pick up blood sugar to put in the cells so it's out of the blood. When blood sugar is normal, insulin is lowered. Once our blood sugar levels out, the barn door closes to keep insulin in.

We can't tell you how many times we've worked with people who've been struggling with their weight and are frustrated. They beat themselves up because they compare themselves to friends who are succeeding and doing the same thing. So then, they decide they just don't have the discipline to lose weight and keep it off and they give up. They lose hope, become depressed and often turn to food (or worse) for comfort, and that is heartbreaking to see. Maybe you've experienced this. The fact is, your inability to lose weight is often due to a decline in your hormones because as we age our hormones get out of balance. Fat STORING hormones get switched on and our fat BURNING hormones like Testosterone, Thyroid and Growth Hormone, are lowered making it difficult to lose weight. It's a health issue.

The Big 5:

There are over 50 hormones in the body—but we want to key in on THE BIG 5 associated with most of the chronic disease epidemic in America today. It's important for you to understand that even if your diet is good and you exercise a lot, your health will suffer if any of these 5 hormones are out of balance.

1. Insulin
2. Thyroid
3. Cortisol
4. Estrogen
5. Testosterone

Let's discuss the organs that secrete these hormones and how they affect your body-

The Pancreas: Stores two hormones that control blood sugar:

1. Insulin: Targets every cell in the body to lower blood sugar by storing it in cells.
2. Glucagon: Targets every cell to increases blood sugar; promotes breakdown of protein and fat.

Let's Start With The BIG KAHUNA- Insulin.

80 million Americans suffer from Insulin Resistance. This is the Colossal Hormone that makes us <u>Sick, Tired, Fat and often Depressed.</u> In excess it causes Inflammation and Chronic Disease. This hormone is like fertilizer for your fat cells. Once you learn how to naturally regulate insulin you will understand how you can shift your body from fat storage to fat-burning. Insulin affects everyone, but some produce a large belly, while other with insulin issues remain thin. Regardless of what happens to your body, the negative effects of insulin on your health are the same. Our bodies produce insulin in response to food, and because insulin is responsible for many processes within our bodies, its critically important for you to have balanced blood sugar, otherwise you will experience the negative effects.

Case Study: Shania

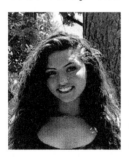

Shania is as 17-year-old female that learned a lot about blood sugar in her junior year of high school due to the stress of college preparation. One day she texted her parents that she felt dizzy, super tired (with the tired face emoji) and lethargic. Her parents asked: "What did you eat today?" "When was your last meal?" After a while she texted them back to tell them she went to the store to get some food and she feels better. Later they asked her what she thought happened and she nailed it when she recounted that she ate mostly carbs for lunch because the protein in her lunch was 'gross'. She stated that school was busy, and she hadn't eaten in over 3 hours. Taking it a step further they asked her what happened in her body— she again nailed it by stating that her blood sugar tanked. A+! She not only corrected her blood sugar, but she understood what caused it to plummet. This is a perfect example of how quickly blood sugar can cause you to malfunction.

Correcting insulin resistance and balancing your blood sugar is well within your reach without medications and the side effects that only band-aid the problems listed here:

Stage 3   Stage 2   Stage 1   Success

- Losing battle with weight, unstable blood sugar increases appetite and sugar craving!
- Increases LDL cholesterol, blood pressure, triglycerides and lowers HDL cholesterol.
- Thickens your blood making it sticky, more likely to clot leading to heart attack and strokes.
- Stimulates cancer cells and increases inflammation
- Prematurely ages your brain and your body.
- Causes infertility and low sex drive by messing with your sex hormones.
- Moodiness . . . After all of this, no kidding!
- Brain degeneration, loss of vision, loss of limbs.

Insulin Balance

You can reset your sugar metabolism to make your cells less insulin resistant by eliminating certain things, while providing nutritional building blocks to restore balance. We address each of our wellness partners differently because everyone is different and unique and may have any number of other issues at play beyond blood sugar issues. Please refer to the end of this chapter and the nutrition chapter for some helpful strategies.

The Thyroid: Produces T4 Thyroxine and T3 triiodothyronine
- Targets every cell in the body to increases the rate of cell metabolism and heart rate

How This Tiny Gland Has Such BIG Implications.

Your thyroid is in charge of how you burn fat and carbohydrates. This is important, because a vicious cycle can develop- as your thyroid worsens so does your blood sugar and in turn your insulin resistance will worsen your thyroid function. So, if your thyroid is low, you can't balance your blood sugar, or your cholesterol, and you can't lose weight. That's why diet, supplements, and optimal thyroid function are critical for metabolism similarly to how you regulate the speed of your car with a gas pedal. Your thyroid is the gas pedal that regulates your metabolism. With the proper setting, your thyroid provides consistent acceleration, thereby allowing optimal metabolism. However, a defective thyroid can decelerate your metabolism (hypothyroidism) or over accelerate (hyperthyroidism), producing heart attacks, diabetes and more. Although some people still associate thyroid problems with classic symptoms of goiter and 'bulging eyeballs,' there are many different symptoms and when they aren't severe or clearly related to the thyroid, healthcare providers often dismiss or blame them on something else.

Common symptoms are:

- Depression, Anxiety, poor concentration, memory
- Weight gain, tired and cold
- PMS, menstrual irregularities, low libido, infertility
- Muscle and joint pain
- Hair loss, course skin, dry mouth, excess ear wax
- Fluid retention, constipation
- High cholesterol, high blood sugar, blood pressure
- Loss of outer eyebrows, loss of ankle reflexes

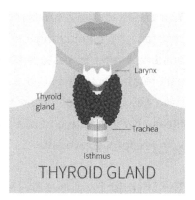

How The Thyroid Gland Functions

1. ONLY 7% of Thyroid hormone is T3, the "active form", which acts on your cells and sends messages to your DNA to turn up metabolism in your mitochondria. T3 is critical to every system in your body to work at the right speed.
2. 93% of what the Thyroid gland produces is a hormone called T4; the 'inactive form' that your body must convert into 'active' T3. Healthy adrenal, liver and stomach function are necessary to convert T4 into active T3. If you produce too little T3, or the T4 is not converted into T3, your metabolism crashes and affects your health.

Do You Have Hypothyroidism?

The first step is to find out if you have symptoms. Thyroid problems are extremely common and even people who have "normal" blood lab tests still suffer from symptoms. It all depends on how we define "normal." As we learn more about the body, the normal values change and what we thought was the norm isn't anymore. For example, for 30 years normal blood pressure was 120/80; now in 2018 it is considered high blood pressure. The same is true with thyroid, cholesterol and even cancer markers over the years, but we can change our approach to thyroid problems by:

*   A Comprehensive Thyroid Assessment: to get the whole picture, seek a functional medicine doctor to order a full comprehensive panel. This will give you far more valuable information than what is covered though insurance.
*   Proper diagnosis results in proper treatment to resolve conditions.
*   Adopt lifestyle changes, diet, and supplements and if necessary, thyroid hormone replacement therapies personally designed for you.

Conventional Insurance Tests Fail

Symptoms are the most important factor in the insurance model, but the tests are only about 30% accurate. It's common to have hypothyroidism and have a normal TSH which is not nearly accurate enough. A functional medicine lab test provides a far more comprehensive picture of your thyroid function to confirm if a sluggish thyroid is contributing to your health issues. There is no one perfect symptom or test. The key is the whole picture—symptoms and blood tests. So, we perform an exam of the thyroid, we look at symptoms and then, we order blood tests. You can start with the Thyroid Questionnaire <u>found on our website member section www. mywellnessmethod.com.</u> If you suspect a sluggish thyroid, ask your doctor to order the **Comprehensive Thyroid Assessment.** This test will reveal thyroid dysfunctions even when TSH and T4 levels are normal. All of this would matter less if thyroid disorders were easily diagnosed and treated, but, they aren't. And here's why:

Hypothyroidism: An Undiagnosed Epidemic

Hypothyroidism is often missed and under-diagnosed because the symptoms are vague and often imitate many other diseases. Consider this; anyone can diagnose a heart attack when we see someone who is pale, sweaty and clutching their chest with pain radiating in the left arm. Thyroid problems are different. Even if you have all the symptoms of low thyroid, they are often overlooked. Even if your doctor orders conventional thyroid tests, often your thyroid appears "normal". Many doctors don't do enough tests so, it goes undetected.

The Comprehensive Thyroid Assessment (CTA) An impressive range of tests available for thyroid function are far more accurate than was possible just five or ten years ago. The **CTA** can detect metabolic irregularities from nutrient deficiencies, toxicity, chronic stress, enzyme malfunction and autoimmune disease even when Thyroid Stimulating Hormone (TSH) and T4 levels are normal. The CTA offers the following results:

- TSH, Free Thyroxine (fT4), Free Triiodothyronine (fT3), Reverse T3, Anti-Thyroglobulin Antibodies, Anti-Thyroid Peroxidase Antibodies, FT4/FT3, FT3/RT3 and adrenal gland function.
- **Central Thyroid Dysregulation** indicates primary or secondary thyroid disease or dysfunction
- **Peripheral Thyroid Dysregulation** nutrient shortages, heavy metal exposure, adrenal stress, enzyme deficiencies, and chronic illness all cause functional hypothyroidism, also known as Euthyroid sick syndrome, low T3 or Wilson's syndrome.
- **Thyroid Antibodies** reveal autoimmune response. Antibodies block thyroid hormones from attaching to cell receptors and cause Hashimoto's thyroiditis, Graves disease or postpartum thyroiditis.

Case Study: Margo

A 54-year-old depressed female struggled with 47% body fat for over ten years. She hired a dietician and a personal trainer and followed their instructions to a T! She was unable to shed the weight and even went so far as to try diet pills. She lost 15 pounds, however, she gained it all back and then some. When she came to see us, we recommended a Comprehensive Thyroid Assessment and found that her peripheral thyroid function (Free T3 and Reverse T3), was abnormal. We recommended our Wellness Method changes and within two months, Margo lost 27 pounds, 4 dress sizes and her symptoms went away. Two years later she is still doing great and holding her weight! Many things contributed to Margo's struggle that we uncovered: diet, stress, environmental toxins, nutrient deficiencies . . . all things that can impact the thyroid. All things YOU can change through a partnership with a reputable functional medicine practitioner! Most doctors don't test thyroid function correctly and many don't address the root cause.

The Important Takeaway Points:

- A Thyroid blood test ordered by her physician told her she **DID NOT** have a thyroid problem.
- Margo's functional lab tests that we performed revealed abnormal peripheral thyroid function (Free T3 and Reverse T3).
- Margo's thyroid would have been overlooked were it not for a thorough thyroid assessment.
- Margo's new lab test showed considerable improvement to match her weight loss.

When Margo came to see us for problems with fatigue, weight gain, poor memory, joint pain and fluid retention, she shared that her doctor's response to her issues was, "Well, what do you expect? You're 54." We recommend you never accept that answer! Your doctor should be like a medical detective who finds clues and puts together the pieces of the story and then works to resolve the underlying cause. In the case of Margo, we tested her for a number of things and found a sluggish thyroid due to an autoimmune reaction. With some simple lifestyle adjustments, she went from feeling old and tired, to vibrant and young again. We see it all the time: Wellness Partners come in with vague complaints that when we put it all together tell an important story. Like anything else, hypothyroidism is not a one-size-fits-all approach. It's important to understand that your thyroid is the master hormone that affects every cell in your body. When it is sluggish, everything slows down.

Preventing Hypothyroidism

Something that has revolutionized our practice has been determining what toxins you've been exposed to, which may be leading to your underproductive thyroid. Then recommend customized nutrients and whole foods that bind to the toxins, and carry them to your liver and kidneys to flush out of your body. It's a sad fact that our food these days lacks the nutrients and minerals that it used to have. The food our great grandparents ate was full of nutrients, vitamins and minerals but in the last hundred years our soil has become denatured and stripped of natural nutrients and our food is full of chemicals. Even if you are eating organic, you still may lack many nutrients. We always test our wellness partners for nutritional deficiencies.

Adrenal Glands - What they do, why they malfunction, and what can you do about it?

Your adrenals help you respond to stress. If you have chronic stress, your adrenals get beat up. A major source of weight-gain is stress. You can actually think yourself fat or thin, and science proves it. Stressful thinking activates metabolic path-ways that cause weight gain and insulin resistance. Remember, stress is a response to stimulation that makes you feel threatened and not always a real circumstance but, rather a perception that you are being attacked. If chronic stress "piles up" it takes a toll physically, mentally and emotionally. The good news is that most stress isn't real. A worry, a thought, or fear of what might go wrong can become intense stress if we carry it with us. If you have survived trauma, it can live in your body even after the stress is gone. Stress is any real or imagined threat and while that might mean fear of a wild animal, it could also mean thinking your spouse, friend or boss is mad at you (even when they aren't).

Stress Hormones

- **Cortisol and Adrenaline** help you run faster, see further, hear better and provide fuel energy to help you survive a threat. This is great in the short term, but prolonged stress and high cortisol elevates blood sugar, belly fat, cholesterol, blood pressure and muscle loss.
- **DHEA** (Dehydroepiandrosterone): is produced by your adrenal glands to balance the effects of cortisol. DHEA has been shown to improve memory, reduce fat storage, improve fat burning and protect you from cell damage caused by aging and disease.

Why Do We Get Adrenal Burnout And How Does It Create Fat?

In healthy people, adrenal glands produce adequate amounts of cortisol and DHEA to help counteract stress. Once the stressful event is over, the adrenal glands have time to 're-charge' but if the stress is allowed to continue, you make too much cortisol to deal with ongoing stress. Elevated cortisol levels lead to insulin resistance which cripples your metabolism. If stress continues over time, the adrenals wear out and can't produce enough cortisol which contributes to an onslaught of health problems. With adrenal burnout, you can't properly respond to stress, so you end up just feeling tired and crummy all the time. You push yourself with coffee or other stimulants to feel better but that only adds more of the same relentless stress of everyday life: stress of work, relationships, finances, stress of always being plugged into the online world.

Runaway Stress Is The Beginning Of Belly Fat: Common signs of Adrenal Burnout:

- You cringe in front of a mirror because of a large belly, loss of muscle and "premature aging."
- You are "tired and wired." Exhaustion rules your day, but you can't sleep.
- Digestive problems and foggy brain are your closest friends.
- Your workouts are, well, not working out!
- Tight muscles cause pain, stiffness and headaches.
- At work, your performance is underwhelming.
- Trouble with low blood pressure or blood sugar.
- Unhealthy, aging skin.
- Craving for salt or sugar.
- You get dizzy when you stand up.
- Depressed.
- You feel overwhelm and your sex drive is gone along with your self-esteem.

So, how do you know if you're on your way to adrenal burnout?

It's very simple. Start by asking yourself the questions on our Adrenal Stress Quiz found on our website member section www. mywellessmethod.com If that confirms adrenal problems the next step is to get tested!

The Adrenal Stress Profile: Science has developed a precise test to help you know how well the adrenal glands are working. Sadly, most doctors order blood lab tests which are not very helpful because cortisol changes throughout the day, so you only get a snapshot at one time of the day, but you are missing the other 24 hours. We do a home test that measures cortisol and DHEA levels all throughout the day.

Eliminating Adrenal Fatigue - The Truth About Managing Your Stress

We don't care how perfect your diet is, if your stress is high, a good diet is cancelled out. Now you might be on a good exercise program too, but if your adrenals are already stressed, exercise only creates MORE STRESS and MORE INFLAMMATION which exacerbates your health condition. Until you lower your stress and heal your adrenal glands you will struggle to lose your belly fat. You must improve your health by lowering your stress. If you'd like to live a fabulous, productive and vital life, then you need to understand that it's not the passing of calendar years that harm you and cause weight gain-its faulty thinking. You can't eliminate stress completely, but you can reduce it with constructive tools to activate pathways that promote weight loss and health. There are all sorts of tools and resources available where you can be guided through the experience.

Case Study: A Note from Judy

As shared earlier, when I met Dr. Kobsar as I hobbled through his clinic doors with a back injury, I was a classic picture of stress. I didn't know I was under stress however, I was just doing my life the way I had always done it. I was artistic director for a dance company in the middle of show production and all that comes with producing high level theatre, I owned a restaurant, a catering business along with my family commitments. Time to take care of myself? I didn't even know what the concept was, it was not vocabulary I had ever heard before. I got sick about 8 times per year- and each time it would take me out of the game for weeks. Still, did I slow down? No, not until I met Dr. Kobsar and his team began to talk to me in a language I had never heard before. Yet I still resisted, because as painful as my back injury was, it was even more painful for me to come to the clinic to get well. I was BUSY! In other words, it was more painful for me to change at first.

Well- they didn't make it optional for me, and slowly they taught me it was critically important to care for myself. In a short amount of time my mind shifted and I became a student of self-care: I dove in and followed Dr. Kobsar's recommendations. It felt odd at first, almost selfish and I had to battle my mind and shift my thinking around this. I had always believed that if I took time for myself then I was a selfish person. All my time should be spent on my daughter, my family, my friends and my work. But as I began to turn the focus towards myself I noticed a fantastic and surprising result! I became a BETTER PERSON *for* my daughter, my family, my friends and my work. I could support them with more strength and clarity than I ever had in my life! Self-care is not selfish, it is one of the most generous things you can do for your loved ones. Begin now to slowly shift towards caring for yourself and watch all the beautiful ways it will manifest in those you love!

Sex Hormones: Estrogen, Testosterone, Progesterone, FSH, LH

"My lack of libido is destroying my relationship. I just feel tired and uninterested in sex. How can I get my mojo back?"

We hear this problem far too often in our practice from those who suffer libido-crashing mood disorders that interfere with their lives. While easy to discount, low sex drive as 'just a part of getting older,' more and more young people are struggling with not being 'in the mood.' Conventional medicine fails to connect the dots between lifestyle and chronic stress, which can contribute to sex hormones being unbalanced. Let's discuss now a few organs that secrete sex hormones and how they affect your body:

The Ovaries:

The ovaries produce two hormones: Estrogen and Progesterone which target sex organs to promote female sex characteristics, store fat and regulate menstrual cycles.

Do you know how ranchers fatten cows before they go to market? **They implant estrogen pellets.** For both genders, too much sugar, refined carbs and alcohol spikes estrogen. Low fiber, and excess antibiotics damage the gut, triggering estrogen spikes because your body can't detoxify properly. Environmental toxins thrive on pesticides which even at low doses act like estrogen. You can bring estrogen into balance by reducing sugar and increasing good fats and fiber. Are you seeing a pattern here? We know that you hear over and over that sugar 'is bad for you', and that you should have a good amount of healthy fats. Now you know WHY these two very simple diet changes are critical for your health. They have so many negative effects on your organs' function, thereby telling your hormones what to do. Make this shift now before you get into real trouble and a doctor recommends hormone replacement therapy!

Weight Gain and Estrogen Dominance

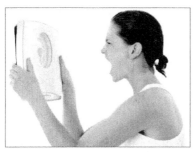
Too much estrogen causes weight gain whether you're a man or a woman. 'Estrogen Dominance' is less related to the amount of circulating estrogen and more related to the ratio of estrogen to progesterone in the body. Excess estrogen, combined with deficient progesterone is the common denominator for female problems that are related to or affected by too much estrogen and too little progesterone. These include:

- Premature aging
- Breast and Uterine cancer
- Muscle and joint pain
- Fat gain in abdomen, hips and thighs
- Hot Flashes
- Hairloss, Bone loss
- Irregular menstrual periods
- Hypoglycemia
- Water retention and bloating

- Autoimmune disorders
- Decreased sex drive
- Depression, Mood swings
- Fatigue, slow metabolism
- Foggy thinking, Memory loss
- Headaches
- Insomnia
- Infertility
- Ovarian fibroid & cysts

* **In men**, it can cause loss of body hair (including chest, legs and arms), a beer belly, low libido, and 'man boobs.'

Causes Of Estrogen Dominance

Besides the hormone fluctuations of menopause, both lifestyle and environment exacerbate estrogen dominance. Estrogen is produced naturally but also in response to substances in our food. We are constantly exposed to petrochemicals and hormones in meat, dairy products, plastic, pollution and medication hormones like the 'The Pill' and Premarin. Sadly, estrogen dominance is a silent epidemic and rarely are women deficient in estrogen; in fact, most are progesterone deficient which gives a balancing effect on estrogen. Supplemental estrogen, even in the slightest amounts, in a woman who doesn't need it, or who has no progesterone to balance it, has many serious side effects.

Women's Bodies Are Not Defective

Sex hormones can drop as much as 90% in women who do not address age related decline. So, are you doomed to suffer from mood swings, bone loss and sexual problems? No, you are not! To think that

75% of women have a design flaw that causes PMS and the need for medical treatment is ridiculous. Simply put, 'female problems' are just imbalanced hormones. They are not the result of poor genes, or bad luck that destroys your sexual vitality as you age. Get your sex hormones in balance and these symptoms will resolve. Your body is not defective: It's lifestyle choices. It comes down to what you do each day and how you live your life in relation to your health. It comes down to your decision to take responsibility or not. YOU have the power to change how your body responds to aging. An 81-year-old wellness partner recently told us, with a twinkle in her eye, about her new boyfriend and their wonderful love life! Thriving is possible at any age without magic pills (which by the way don't exist).

The Most Comprehensive Hormone Test Women Need

The typical hormone tests ordered by most doctors include Luteinizing Hormone (LH), follicle-stimulating hormone (FSH), estradiol (E2). Unfortunately, this is **NOT** adequate to determine if you are suffering with estrogen dominance. We offer a comprehensive female hormone panel that includes: E2 (estradiol), 1 (Estrone) and E3 (Estriol), Progesterone, 2-Hydroxyestrone (good estrogen) and 16-alpha Hydroxyestrone (bad estrogen). You need a ratio for 2: 16 alpha Hydroxyestrone. This optimal ratio should be greater than . 40. This test tells if you are truly Estrogen Dominant.

The Testes

The testes produce Testosterone which targets ovaries, breasts, testes and muscles by traveling through your blood to assist in the development of female and male sex characteristics. Some common symptoms of low testosterone include:

- Weight gain, loss of vigor
- Infertility and loss of sex drive

- Heart disease
- Depressed and Irritable or impatient with loved ones
- Accelerated and Premature aging
- Loss of muscle mass

The #1 Killer Of Sex Drive

Testosterone isn't just a guy's hormone—women need it too! In both men and women, it can reduce desire, increase body fat, lower muscle mass and accelerate aging. Lack of exercise, alcohol, stress, toxins or pituitary conditions lower testosterone leading to erectile dysfunction, low sex drive, fatigue, brain fog and bone loss that leads to osteoporosis, so it is clear that getting and keeping testosterone levels up naturally is a priority for you whether you are a male or female.

Testosterone Tests Fall Short

A consistent finding in the scientific studies is that obese men have low testosterone and high estrogen. Once again we find that 'normal ranges' found in the insurance-based lab results are not optimal for those wanting to lose weight and increase sex drive. If you are a man over age 40 and your physician tells you that your testosterone is 'normal,' it does not mean that your testosterone and estrogen are in optimal, youthful ranges, because remember- 'normal' ranges come from the average of all the people that go to that lab. Wouldn't you want your ranges to be optimal? The optimal range is where fat loss will naturally occur.

Beware of testosterone replacement therapy - it comes with many risks and if you are considering this, have a prostate-specific antigen (PSA) blood test and digital rectal exam to rule out prostate cancer. Most times you have the ability to naturally balance your testosterone levels and without testosterone medications.

CASE STUDY: George

George was pre-diabetic and struggled with his weight, his cholesterol, had chronic pain for 15 years and had lost his sex drive. He tried a cleanse diet, the paleo, the ketogenic, and was very vigilant in following them. We put him on a low-sugar, whole-foods diet plan with plenty of healthy fats and supplements and we addressed lifestyle factors. Within 4 months he lost 53 pounds and his libido recharged because sex hormone imbalances are often the result of more serious health problems. For example: Cholesterol is needed to produce testosterone and other sex hormones. Eating a low-fat diet and taking statin drugs block cholesterol production which can negatively alter your sex hormones. Another example is too much sugar raises insulin which may lower testosterone. So, a healthy sex drive requires a reduction of sugar intake. When you balance insulin and cholesterol, sex hormones often fall into place and optimize the libido. If you suspect imbalances, go get tested for imbalances by a functional medicine practitioner. More strategies to increase sex drive are covered at the end of this chapter.

Take our Sex Hormone Quiz <u>found on our website member section</u> <u>www.mywellnessmethod.com</u> Remember that the best way to know if you have an imbalance is a blood test, but the quiz results give you a good place to start to reveal imbalances.

Healing Your Endocrine System

Many of us are taught that high blood sugar is not reversible, but this has been proven wrong many times over. Don't wait to go blind, lose limbs, suffer strokes or toxic liver failure from medications! One study entitled "<u>Reversal of type 2 diabetes: normalization of</u> <u>beta cell function in association with decreased pancreas and liver</u> <u>triglycerides</u>" showed a change in diet without exercise reversed most signs of diabetes within one week and all features by eight weeks. That's right, DIABETES WAS REVERSED IN ONE WEEK! That's more powerful than any drug known to modern medicine. Another groundbreaking study showed that even people with a damaged pancreas can recover. When you make the changes your blood sugar will lower, triglycerides drop, and your pancreas recovers. So despite what you might hear, there is hope. Let's talk about what you can do today to begin restoring your hormone balance.

1. **First, take our quiz** on our website to see what, if you have symptoms of hormone imbalance.

2. **Find a Reputable Functional Medicine Practitioner to Test and Interpret Your Labs.** It's important to get the correct lab tests by going outside of the insurance system. Remember, invest in yourself and the return will be your health and vitality long after you write the check.

3. **Metabolic Assessment** reveals your metabolic age, your cellular health, hydration and body composition.

4. **Avoid Hormone Replacement Therapy!** For 50 years estrogen therapy was thought to be the 'fountain of youth' until it was found that it increased uterine cancer eight-fold. For more than three decades, this kind of hormone therapy created unnecessary harm through increases in uterine, breast, ovarian cancer, heart attacks and strokes. These methods provide a temporary fix to symptoms.

HEALING AND BALANCING ACTION STEPS

If lab tests confirm your quiz results, it's time to put a plan to action. Remove toxins that start the problem, heal the organs that produce hormones, provide the nutrients needed to construct hormones and begin certain exercises to KICK START your glands to produce fat burning, anti-aging hormones. Understand that everyone is different, and guidance from a qualified practitioner always yields the best results.

Here are some action steps to get started:

Action Step 1: Liver and Stomach Repair
If your liver detoxification system isn't working, this is important to address. Use the action steps in the inflammation chapter to restore your stomach health which helps your hormones.

Action Step 2: Chill-ax. Turn down the stress hormones of aging and fat storing!
Find something to reduce your stress. Meditation, yoga, a creative outlet . . . find some things you like to hit your pause button. Lowering stress doesn't sound sexy, but it's oh so necessary in our fast-paced culture. Stress leads to disease and causes more stress so get a handle on stress or it will handle YOU.

A certain amount of healthy stress is fine, it keeps us moving forward and growing, but you must reduce unwanted stress immediately. Make a list of the most stressful people and circumstances in your life and make a plan to mitigate the effects on you. Use these suggestions and more from the coaching chapter of this book:

- **List the most intense stressors in your life** starting with 1, 2, 3 and so on.
- **Focus on the biggest stress first.** Get clear on why it causes stress. Be honest here, even if its uncomfortable because if you just gloss over the 'why', you can't move to the next step.

- **List 3 action steps you can take to minimize stress.** Notice we said, 'action steps that YOU can take'. We didn't say, "3 action steps the other person can do." This is about you. No one can make you feel a certain way without your permission to let them.
- **Actions steps aren't easy . . .** if they were you probably would've taken them already. Take small steps every day. If you fall back, get up and go again.

Action Step 3: Sleep

Your body has the best chance of recovery from stress if you go to bed by 10PM. Physical repair takes place between approximately 10PM and 2AM. Your immune cells patrol your body eliminating cancer cells, bacteria, viruses, etc. . . . Then from 2AM to 6AM, your brain gets re-charged, releasing chemicals that enhance your immune system. So, if you find that you are not getting to bed until 12AM, you have just robbed your body of two solid hours of healing. At least seven to eight hours of uninterrupted sleep every night is one of the best ways to balance hormones. Studies show "even one night of poor sleep can increase insulin resistance"--- The Endocrine Society's Journal of Clinical Endocrinology & Metabolism. Sleep hygiene is crucial so finding a quality mattress and pillow is helpful and so is avoiding electronic devices before bed. Use aromatherapy and music to set the mood for sleep and reserve your bedroom only for sleep and intimacy with your partner.

ACTION STEP 4: Move more

Adopt a comprehensive, personalized exercise plan as described in the exercise chapter. When you exercise properly, you affect insulin, cortisol, thyroid and sex hormones in a positive way. Get out in the fresh air to get natural light to affect your pineal gland to reset your stress response.

Action Step 5: Rhythm Method

We also recommend a regular routine. Rhythm is key, because your hormones follow balanced rhythms. So, exercise at the same time daily, go to bed at the same time, eat at the same time - rhythms in life help restore balance. Take breaks when you are tired. Our bodies function best on what we call "Rhythm Method" which is cycles of 90 minutes of activity punctuated by a few minutes of rest or zoning out.

ACTION STEP 6: Assess the Toxins in Your Home

Cleaning Supplies: Look through your cleaning supplies and you will find most of them are full of harmful chemicals. There are many natural cleaning product lines that you can replace those dangerous products with. One we like is Doterra but there are others. You can look into these products here: https://www.doterra.com/US/en/site/wellnessmethod

Body-care products- Toothpaste, hair products, soaps, lotions, creams . . . you get the picture. We are literally slathering harmful chemicals onto our bodies every day. 75% of estrogen for women and 50% of adult testosterone for is made in the skin AND so is 100% of post-menopausal estrogen! The skin my friends IS an endocrine (hormone) organ, and the biggest one we have. The skin makes hormones including IGF-1, Thyroid and Human Growth Hormone so, the chemicals you put on your skin, go through this hormone factory. Everything from metabolic syndrome, diabetes, heart disease, cancer . . . are linked to hormones in the skin. Your skin and brain are close friends having come from the same fetal tissues and the skin is constantly feeding data to the brain based on what it absorbs, and your brain changes your body chemistry in response. **Want to improve your testosterone or estrogen?** Protect your skin from chemicals in laundry products, cosmetics, fragrances, etc.

ACTION STEP 7: Avoid the Dirty Dozen Hormone Disruptors: (courtesy of the Environmental Working Group.)

- **BPA (plastics)** - imitates estrogen causing breast and other cancers, reproductive problems, heart disease, early puberty, etc. Avoid paper receipts coated in BPA, plastics labelled "PC," for polycarbonate, or recycling label #7 and canned goods—or research the companies using BPA in products.
- **Atrazine (insecticide)** Widely used on corn and in drinking water. Linked to breast tumors, delayed puberty and prostate cancer. Buy organic produce and a water filter certified to remove atrazine.
- **Phthalates**, can cause birth defects, obesity, diabetes, thyroid problems and sperm count. Avoid plastic food containers, children's toys and plastic wrap made from PVC with the recycling label #3. Also avoid personal care products that list added "fragrance."
- **Perchlorate (Chlorines)** It competes with thyroid hormones. Use a reverse osmosis filter. Impossible to avoid in food but Iodine reduces its effects.
- **Lead** causes permanent brain damage, miscarriage, high blood pressure, kidney damage, diabetes, anxiety, depression and disrupts stress hormones. Avoid crumbling old paint and get a good water filter.
- **Arsenic** causes cancer of the skin, bladder and lungs, obesity, disrupts blood sugar, muscles loss, depressed immunity, diabetes, osteoporosis, growth retardation and high blood pressure. Get a water filter that lowers arsenic. Look into a water filter we recommend https://www.aquatruwater.com?src=affiliate&aid=45890

- **Mercury** interferes with brain development in a fetus, women's menstrual cycles and damages the pancreas. AVOID wild salmon and farmed trout.
- **PFC's (Per fluorinated Chemicals)** Affects thyroid and sex hormones, kidney disease, thyroid disease and birth weight. Avoid non-stick cookware, stain resistant coatings on clothing, furniture and carpets.
- **Polybrominated Diphenyl Ethers PBDE's:** These Fire Retardants imitate thyroid hormones. Use a vacuum cleaner with a HEPA filter and take care when reupholstering foam furniture or replacing the padding under old carpets.
- **Organophosphate Pesticides** lowers testosterone and thyroid hormones. Buy organic fruit and veggies.
- **Glycol Ethers:** Found in paint solvents, cleaning products, brake fluid and cosmetics. Lowers sperm count and children have more asthma and allergies. Avoid 2-butoxyethanol (EGBE) and methoxydiglycol (DEGME).
- **Dioxin** (insecticide) Disrupts male and female sex hormones and affects sperm. Powerful carcinogen that affects your immune system. Eat fewer animal products.

ALIGNMENT OF YOUR STRUCTURE

Regimen
Educational Curriculum
Coaching
Reducing Inflammation
Endocrine System
Alignment of Your Structure
Total Nutrition
Exercise

*The doctor of the future will give no medication, but
will interest his patients in the care of the human frame,
diet and in the cause and prevention of disease."*

~ *Thomas A. Edison*

How Your Structural Alignment Keeps You in Sync
*"Your body is in a constant state of change, and while we
do a lot of things right, the average American lifestyle
perpetuates premature aging, breakdown and destruction of
the structure, including the nervous system. The daily rigors
of life are enough to wreak havoc on our structural health
from the way we work to the way we play- we ask a lot of our
bodies. But when you can implement and perpetuate positive*

change, give yourself support and enhancement, you will then be on the path to sustaining proper nervous, muscular and skeletal system function for years. Let's take a look at the reasons why we get out of sync over time in order to understand how to find our way back to structural health".

~ Dr. Kobsar's article,
Pathways to Family Wellness, August 2017.

Postural Structuring Begins In The Womb

How did I get like this? What should I have done differently? These are questions you might be asking and these are questions we hear from our wellness partners in our office every day. There are several reasons why we end up out of balance. Genetic coding plays a role when you are in your mother's womb, because the fetus and the nutritional environment provided by the mother orchestrates our structural development. Amniotic fluid pressure and other soft tissue intra-uterine pressures begin to contribute to your posture or relative positioning of all your body parts once developed. Intrauterine positioning and your size as a fetus have been related to musculo-skeletal development that will play an important role when you learn to walk.

Postural Structuring After Birth

"Head forward posture can add up to 30 pounds of abnormal leverage on the cervical spine. Forward Head Posture may result in the loss of 30 per cent of vital lung capacity."

~ Rene Cailliet,
MDDirector of Physical Medicine and Rehabilitation,
University Southern California

If your physical structure takes form in the womb, then your restructuring takes place from birth on. Your progressive strengthening and straightening of your posture from what was observed at birth will now be dictated by your environment. Two important factors that will dictate this are your body mass and gravity. By the time your body is less than half of your adult size, you have already learned to perform complex postural maneuvers. Even before you finish growing (age 14-18), you may have reached the best body posture of your life, yet after age 18 your posture will begin to decline. At this point you may experience a general weakening of the soft tissue which accompanies the destructive-postural changes; this stimulates fat deposition that can sometimes conceal the changes in your posture.

From ages 25-45 the gradual degradation of posture continues with many associated health problems and obvious signs associated with the aging process. From age 45 until death, destructive postural changes become obvious with inward rotation of the legs and increased curvature of the spine. These postural changes may result in as much as a 1 and 1/2 inch decrease in height by the time we are in our 30's and we will continue to lose several inches until we die. Conventional exercise can contribute to your postural decline as well. It's too hard on your body and it accelerates aging of your joints. Right now, you may be beating yourself up for not exercising more, but what's more important than 'how often you exercise' is 'HOW you exercise'.

If you're over 60 we know that you may be worried about retiring with a body that's riddled with illness or pain. We want you to ENJOY your golden years with energy and health, so that is why it's so important for you to understand how and why your posture and your structure declines and find out how to create the body you can thrive with into your golden years. That is what this chapter is all about, so get ready to learn how to align and maximize your structure for a vital life! The alternative is to gain weight, become sedentary, and start producing inflammatory molecules that create an environment in your body of chronic pain. When muscles become inactive they cease to do their job to support your joints causing muscular imbalance: this leads to injuries. If one side is weak you may appear to function normally until the wrong motion causes the inevitable injury. Imbalanced muscles cause joint and muscle pain and accelerate arthritis due to the wear and tear that results.

Is Deteriorating Posture An Inevitable Part Of Aging?

Logic would tell you that posture progressively deteriorates in all of us as we age. In fact, anyone who might dare suggest otherwise would rightfully be viewed with a lot of skepticism. Even though the importance of good posture has been recognized and depicted in the writings and drawings of many ancient civilizations, we pay little attention to reversing the postural changes associated with aging.

What Causes Poor Posture As We Age?

Most scientists will tell you it is gravity, and we agree. Physics teaches us that Force = Mass x Acceleration. The acceleration of gravity multiplied by our body weight equals the force that pulls posture towards the ground. Gravity obviously remains constant but as you age and accumulate more body mass, the force on your structure increases. By the time most you reach the age of 14 the force that must be supported by your legs is too great, and posture begins to breakdown. Gravity pronates the foot, tilts your pelvis forward and increases spinal curves. These destructive changes in posture are explained by this basic law of physics. Postural changes can cause pain in many people if not addressed and corrected. Pain left unattended can send you down a road riddled with medications and mental suffering.

America's Pain Crisis

The sad lesson of Tom Petty symbolizes what so many others suffer with when it comes to pain. The overdose death of musician Tom Petty reflects the combination of prescription pain pills and ongoing pain that has killed so many. When we are dealing with injured people, we are dealing with very fragile people. Even the super successful, like the man who wrote "Running Down a Dream", "An American Girl" and "I Won't Back Down"- had human frailties. He was the classic American success story, overcoming humble beginnings by sticking to a plan, working hard and rising above adversity only to end with an accidental overdose of pain medication used for a broken hip during a concert tour. Petty kept his band together for decades and even fought the powerful music industry to win artistic freedom and music rights. Unfortunately, like many, he carried mental health challenges. He helped others with his willingness to publicly discuss his battle with depression - which nearly always accompanies a physical injury, and all of us are susceptible.

Pain Care Strategies

- **First Thought**; I have pain
- **Second Thought:** Which medication should I take?

Before you can move into reprogramming your structural alignment, you must reduce all joint and muscle pain and unfortunately too many people are using a failed approach. With all the new data, the medical community is SLOWLY starting to move away from pain drugs. In February 2017, the American College of Physicians advised doctors to prescribe "non-drug therapies" such as exercise and chiropractic for pain, and avoid drugs or surgery wherever possible. In March 2016, the Centers for Disease Control issued guidelines urging doctors to use non-drug options but America has a long way to go. Opioids remain rampant across the US and in 2018, the epidemic has only gotten worse. The first step is awareness. We must wake up and think differently about pain care.

Chronic pain is defined as pain that persists longer than the natural healing recovery period associated with a disease or injury. It's good to remember that pain is subjective and only the person experiencing the pain knows how it truly feels. Pain perception involves both the central nervous system and the peripheral nervous system. The nerves of the peripheral nervous system convey messages to the brain via the spinal cord. When persistent pain transmission occurs, a-wind up phenomenon induces a change that allows pain signals to transmit more easily. This change may even hijack non-pain nerves and get them to transmit pain signals as well. Chronic pain can cause depression, anxiety and less physical activity leading to degeneration, hormone imbalance and accelerated aging.

Simple Pain and Complex Pain

We can understand the essence of pain better when we look at it and break it down into simple pain and complex pain. This allows us to see that some problems won't be solved by quick fixes like turmeric or pain medications.

1. **Simple Pain**: is a purely structural problem. It has a simple cause that has a simple solution that we like to call the **Base Stealers.** Examples of simple pain are outlined in this table:

Simple Injury	Simple Cause	Simple Solution
Muscle pain	Poor posture or car accident	Correct the posture. Treat and strengthen damaged muscles.
Joint pain	Ruptured a knee ligament	Repair the rupture, heal the injury, strengthen the joint.

Simple pain care incorporates the **Base Stealers** which is the standard of care found in most orthopedic, chiropractic or physical therapy clinics. It consists of 4 steps:

1. Reduce inflammation: ice, electrotherapies, topical creams, etc.
2. Improve mobility/flexibility/range of motion: chiropractic adjustments, massage, stretching, foam rollers, etc.
3. Strengthen weakened and injured muscles. Resistance training with TheraBand's, free weights, nautilus machines, etc.
4. Correct Posture: This is the missing step in more than 70 percent of rehabilitation clinics that focus only on the injured joints but ignore the kinetic chain that runs through your structure. It is critical for long term improvement.

2. **Complex Pain:** Goes beyond only structural concerns so we need the **'Big Hitters'**. It will not be resolved by a simple pain care approach because it involves many systems of the body that malfunction. Pain with these conditions must be addressed by interventions that use a global approach—*the* **'Big Hitters'** *on the team. But we still need the* **'Base Stealers'** *like improving posture or core strengthening.*

Complex Injury	Complex Causes	Complex Solution
Muscle and Joint pain	Poor posture, car accident, sports injury	Treat the damaged muscles and ligaments. Correct the posture
Immune system, endocrine system, nervous system.	diabetes, depression, autoimmune disease, chronic fatigue, etc.	Diet, anti-inflammatory lifestyle changes, sleep, exercise, stress management, detoxification.

Complex Pain Care: A one cause, one solution approach won't work here. When you have joint or muscle pain, it feels like the fix should come from the area where the pain is present. But in complex pain we often work on systems that are distant from your pain sensation. You can't chase complex pain, you must correct the system malfunction or risk a life of crippling pain and dependence on canes, walkers or wheel chairs. This can severely affect interactions with your children, grandchildren, and not to mention intimacy with your spouse/partner because everything hurts.

Systems Not Structures

Since complex pain is often unrelated to tissue damage but rather to things like an inflammatory lifestyle, obesity, anxiety and depression, blood sugar, diet, toxins and insomnia to name a few - you must address the systems, including the Gastrointestinal, Hormones, Nervous, etc. As an example, here are some changes that happen with hormones and neurotransmitters:

Increased When Pain is Reduced	Increased When Pain is Increased
Dopamine	Cortisol
Oxytocin	Insulin
Serotonin	Relaxin
Endorphins	Prenenelone
Adrenaline	Estrogen
Testosterone	

How Complex Pain Compromises Your Mind and Body

Complex pain can last for months, years or decades and compromise every aspect or your life. Your systems are shifted to higher or lower levels of sensitivity. For the sensitive person, whenever there is stress, there is a strong response. This person may feel pain, fatigue or weakness to even a minor stress. While others have a system that remains strong in the face of significant stress. They can run a marathon, be in a car accident, work 80 hours/week, and go about life with no dip in energy and vitality.

It's good to know your level of stress tolerance, so you can have better judgment about your ability to cope with stress. Knowing your pain and fatigue is not 'all in your head' helps you intelligently manage your stress. Tolerance levels can easily change for the worse—severe trauma can cause a phase shift in our systems, making them hyper reactive. But hyper reactive systems can shift back to a normal set point through rest, stress management and improving general health. Unfortunately, this usually doesn't happen overnight.

Here is what a compromised life looks like:

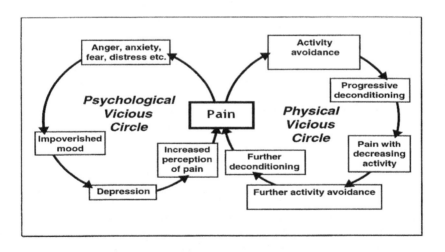

- You're trying to cope with a loss of your job since you can no longer work, and you are on disability.
- Financial worries that follow your job loss.
- Chronic (complex) pain makes you irritable with loved ones.
- which leads to anxiety and depression.

- Days are filled with doctor's appointments, hospital admissions, procedures.
- Endless medications causing addiction and toxicity of your stomach liver and kidneys resulting in more medications.
- Affects your marriage, time spent with children and grandkids.
- Your golden years are spent struggling and suffering instead of travelling and enjoying these years of life.

Don't worry, you are almost there! We have to teach you how the body declines before we teach you how to restore! Remember, education is key to recreating your health through our Wellness Method.

The 4 Pain Generators: The 4 pain generators of the structural system are:

1. Immobile or Stuck Joints
2. Dys-coordinated muscle contraction causing trigger points, muscle tightness
3. The Nervous System
4. Emotions and Mental health

Things often start so innocently as pain gradually begins to increase and it's all too easy to dismiss because it sneaks up slowly. Yet, just like any disease that moves slowly (tooth decay, heart disease, cancer) pain is often pushed aside until the damage is irreversible. So whether you've had physical trauma or not, we all accumulate damage to some degree. Your structure undergoes physical stress every day that creates damage. Add the assaults of chemical stress and emotional stress and you've got a recipe for degeneration. But in this chapter, we are focused on attention to your structure so let's get started learning how to do that!

Structural Reset - The 3 Superhero Systems

Here is our proven path to hit Reset on your structure at any age. There are 3 systems in your body that misfire or shut down and they are the root cause of structural disease. The degeneration of these 3 systems will ravage your body by attacking your joints, muscles and bones, and affects how fast you age structurally. The good news is, you can leverage the power of your body's ability to 'reset' by moving smart and putting these 3 systems to work FOR you. Structural Reset slows the compensation of pain movement patterns. Since our structure functions as one system, any injury causes a kinetic chain of events throughout your body called an adaptive response or more simply 'it compensates'. We created 'Structural Reset' because too many people over the age of 35 are still going about things the hard way:

- Dangerous and addictive pain medication
- Endless doctor's appointments and specialists
- Ongoing Physical Therapy and Massage therapy visits
- 'Magic Pill' supplements, herbs and natural remedies

But if you reset your 3 Structural Superheroes, you can restore your structure to the prime of your life! We've been guiding people through our proven Structural Reset method for over 20 years. The stories we hear every day from our wellness partners across the country are not 'ordinary' stories of success!

- Retirees and Empty Nesters return to their prime, enjoying newfound "drive" and getting back into a spirit of play.

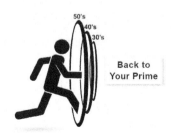

50's
40's
30's

Back to
Your Prime

- Busy Parents from all walks of life are enjoying prime-of-life energy that reminds them of when they were youngsters, bounding about in a playful state of optimism and excitement.

You can switch back on your 3 Structural Superheroes regardless of your age, so don't go down the road of, "I'm too old". We call these 3 structural superhero systems your Structural Priming Activators (SPA's). Your SPA's worked naturally when you were in your prime, but you can reset them. Remember the days when you could exercise <u>without</u> having to worry about paying for it the next day? Or when you could move more freely <u>without</u> feeling muscle aches or inflamed and swollen joints? Adolescent bodies are **protected** by SPA's. Why? Because we moved all the time. When we stopped moving, these 3 systems went into dysfunctional mode. The result: these joint-supporting, muscle-protective systems vanish as we age. For many, your structure has aged too fast. The good news is it can be "time-warped" back to the days:

- When you slept like a baby.
- When you could go for a hike without fearing the repercussions.
- When sitting for a couple hours on a plane or in a car did not require a strategic plan
- When you picked up your kids and threw them in the air as they giggled and screamed with joy
- **When you felt more <u>alive</u>.**

When these systems were first discovered, researchers viewed them as gifts of youth, but they were wrong! In the late 2000s, scientists connected the dots between motion and the 3 systems. It turns out that it wasn't "youth" that was driving the positive effects of SPA's, but rather specific ways of moving that we do naturally when we are in our prime. Taking this research, we created a 'youth cocktail'- a specific system of structural movements custom designed for folks over the age of 35. Structural Reset re-awakens dormant 'muscles' and resets the SPAs that return you to your prime.

Structural Reset: Your 3 Superhero SPA's

"Good posture can be successfully acquired only when the entire mechanism of the body is under perfect control".

~ Joseph Pilates

The 3 'Superhero SPA's' of Structural Reset are signaling agents that "talk" to your structure. Think of SPA's as a structural drill sergeant barking orders to your brain, muscles, and joints, and forcing them to obey every command and train them to work on auto-pilot. These 3 superhero SPA's serve a specific function and Structural Reset harnesses those functions to work for you. The 3 SPA's that protect you are:

1. Muscle Balance
2. Joint Alignment
3. The Nervous System

1. MUSCLE BALANCE—Superhero #1:

Your structure consists of bones, joints, ligaments, muscles and other tissues that protect you. In the diagram we see perfect balance. The red muscles are pulling on the black bones

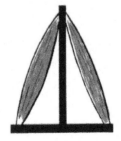

equally from each side. Injury happens when muscles get over loaded, over-stretched, torn, or repeated stressed. This irritates them and triggers a protective mechanism that deactivates injured muscles for their own protection, much like a 'blown circuit.' Until the muscle nerve is reset or rebooted, the muscle remains inactive. As you move thru daily life activities, other muscles must compensate for the inactive muscle causing an increase of nerve impulses to that muscle. If nerve impulses are too low or too high, it causes pain, numbness, tingling, spasm, weakness, etc. All of which has consequences, starting with the debilitating path to degeneration unless injuries are corrected.

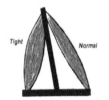

That's right! That lifting injury you had 15 years ago that hurts you when the weather changes, may be the underlying cause of your constipation or adrenal hormone imbalance. How can this be? The nerve malfunction caused by the injury affects the colon's mobility and causes constipation. You may try all types of remedies from fiber, a colon cleanse or even a colonoscopy that shows no problems. If the nerve is not restored, the function of your internal system will be impaired. The good news is that we are made up of cells and tissue that have the ability to recover and heal. If the nerve is reset and nerve impulses restored, better function will usually follow.

Signs of Impaired Muscle Balance:

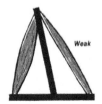

1. Tight or weak muscles.
2. Joints are out of alignment.
3. Muscles that are 'too slow' or 'too fast'.

When A Muscle Is Activated (The Agonist), The "Antagonist (Opposing) Muscle" Must Be Inhibited.

- Tight low back extensor. The muscles that arch your low back are called 'extensors.' If they are tight, you can't fully contract your abdominal muscles. Why? Because the abdominals are the Antagonist (opposing) muscles to the extensors, and when the extensors are tight they pull the abdominals away from their position of strength and can't fire properly.
- Tight biceps. The muscles that bend your elbow are called 'biceps'. If they are tight then you can't fully contract your triceps muscles. Why? Because the triceps are the Antagonist (opposing) muscles to the biceps, and when the biceps are tight they pull the triceps away from their position of strength and can't fire properly.

Solution: Remove the muscle stress of the hyperactive muscle or it will remain activated. More on this later in the chapter.

You can learn more about the science behind this by studying the three types of nerves that are responsible:

- Alpha nerves cause muscle contraction.
- Gamma nerves cause muscles to lengthen/stretch.
- Golgi Tendons sets the parameters of balance.

2. JOINT ALIGNMENT—Superhero #2:

The average American lifestyle is grossly deficient in movement which is needed to fire nerves in your joints to stimulate your brain and spinal cord, so it's not surprising that you need periodic alignment resets. Without periodic alignments, your joints tend to freeze-up and fewer nerve receptors fire and the power nerve impulses needed to energize your nervous system diminish. Managing joint degeneration and alignment restores motion so joint receptors fire correctly. Misalignment creates an unbalanced distribution of force and causes:

1. Joint swelling, muscle spasm and pain.
2. Premature Joint Degeneration (osteoarthritis).
3. Stuck joints cause excess motion in nearby joints to compensate.
4. Altered joint balance receptors result in compensations that reprogram the nervous system.

Your body compensates for pain by restricting your joints with tight muscles, calcification, neuropathy and so forth. Before long, everything seems normal again because you no longer feel pain. After all, they aren't moving, but here's the problem. This is planting the seed for 'arthritis' or 'degenerative joint disease'. So, over the course of 5-10 years, your joint disease gets worse, much like rusting of metal. It leaves corrosion around the nerves that are supposed to fire in your spine to keep it powered up. The longer the damage, the less energy available for the nervous system. Nerve impulses are reduced, and degeneration leads to disc disease, bone spurs, pain and neuropathy. All of these affect communication to your brain and overall health.

Why Alignment Matters

*"The beginning of the disease process
begins with postural distortions."*

~ Hans Selye, Nobel Laureate

Joint misalignment is the most common place for nerve system interference. If your spine gets out of alignment, the vertebrae act as resistors to the distribution of your nervous system energy. *"Misalignments interfere with the flow of nerve impulses and it only takes pressure as light as a quarter (10mm/hg) for three minutes to reduce nerve function by 60%. Nerve degeneration literally begins within hours."* -- Dr. Suh, University of Colorado neurophysiologist.

Solution: Joint alignment can be restored by an alignment and the foremost experts here in America are chiropractors. Balancing your muscles will help the alignment hold longer but it will not release a frozen joint that is stuck in place.

THE NERVOUS SYSTEM—Superhero #3

"The nervous system controls and coordinates all organs and structures of the human body."

~ Gray's Anatomy Textbook

The Nervous System is your "Master Computer". Your brain is the control center of every function in your body. If your brain dies, you die. As long as your brain can communicate with every organ, tissue and cell of your body, you have the potential for healing and optimal health. Your nervous system—coordinates all communication. Nerve impulses from the brain travel down the spinal tract to signal nerves to activate muscles. In order to move, your brain contracts your muscles. The left brain controls the muscles on the right side of your body and the right brain controls the left side. In other words, your spine is the freeway from your brain to the level of your spine that connects to a muscle (motor) nerve which signals the muscle to contract. This process controls posture, core muscles and movements.

The Brain and spinal cord control your **Autonomic (automatic) Nervous System** which supplies nerve impulses to blood vessels, organs and glands. It receives and responds to information about your body from two divisions:

- <u>Sympathetic:</u> - Stimulates overall body functions
- <u>Parasympathetic:</u> - Lowers overall body functions

Your Autonomic Nervous System controls many body processes:

- Blood pressure, heart rate and breathing
- Digestion, Metabolism and body temperature
- Body fluids (saliva, sweat, mucous and tears)
- Urination and Bowel movements
- Sexual function

Why is this important? Because your Autonomic system responds to stress by increasing sympathetic nervous-system activity causing hyperactivity, stomach issues, fatigue, heart problems, etc. If the stress is 'perceived' to be prolonged you pay the price.

How Alignment of Your Spine Affects Your Autonomic Nervous System

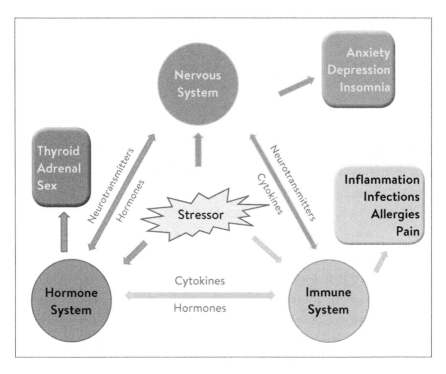

Your brain sends 100% of your body's information and energy down your spinal cord which is protected by your vertebrae. Spinal nerves exit between vertebrae to deliver the messages from your brain to each cell, muscle and organ of your body. And through the same system, messages are returned so that you can function at your best. But if nerve restrictions suppress or garble these messages, your body will not be able to do what it was programmed to do—heal itself. It will not be *able* to execute its built-in, self-healing program. Therefore, interference in your nervous system creates health problems.

Nervous System Interference

"Proper posture sends a positive message since 90% of all communication occurs through body language and how you carry yourself."

~ *Cindy Ann Peterson*

Interference in your nervous system creates Interference in all your body systems and affects your body function. Your brain monitors and responds to stress in your body. It regulates thirst, hunger, body temperature, blood pressure, etc., by linking the nervous system to the hormone system by the 'negative feedback loop' we discussed earlier . . . here's another example: An intruder breaks into your home. When your brain perceives that danger, the brain fires a nerve impulse to trigger the fight-or flight response, which stimulates the adrenal glands to release cortisol, to aid in your survival. Once the threat is removed, the brain has the job of *reversing* all the biological stress created because it is no longer needed so, it signals the nervous system to calm things back to normal. Problems arise when our brain senses we are in constant stress because the negative feedback loop system fails and keeps running. The results are degeneration and an ongoing breakdown of your nerve system and physical body.

Let's pause a moment here because you are gaining a lot of critically valuable insights of how your body breaks down, ages, contracts pain and disease. It is undeniable that if you do not understand how the body protects itself, then you will never gain an understanding of how to heal. If all we presented here for you are a bunch of quick fixes, it would only help temporarily. Understanding the origin of disease and pain and the steps to optimal health is the only path to gaining true independence. Can you put a price tag on your life? You are the ONLY you on the planet. Your life's value is priceless to you, to your family and therefore the education you are getting is vital. It is beyond value because it's critical for *your life* for as long as you live. What has more value than that?

The education here should be in the hands of school age kids from the moment they begin their health education. Our schools don't teach this and it is vital to educate our children from a young age about their health—their most precious asset! So we feel passionate about the education we provide here and will not stop until there is a shift in how our society views 'healthcare'. Our hope is that you not only learn these principles, but that you pass them on your kids, your grandkids, your loved-ones. Pay it forward to family and friends. Be our partners in our mission to change the way we understand and care for our lives. Now, let's continue learning how the 'control center' of your body aides in your recovery.

How to Reboot, Reset and Restore your 3 Super Hero's

Muscle Balance, Joint Alignment and Nervous System

Movement is the key to "Reboot" your nervous system. Dr. Roger Sperry, Nobel Prize winner for brain research discovered that our brain and spinal cord must be perpetually stimulated to stay powered up. But how do we stimulate it? After all, we don't plug ourselves in every night to recharge so what powers your systems? Dr. Sperry discovered tiny receptors in your spinal joints that fire whenever they move, sending impulses to the brain and spinal cord much like a motion-powered watch works. The watch has no battery but has an internal rotor that reacts to movement of your wrist. As the rotor turns, it winds the watch to store power to run the watch. Without movement, the watch will stop. This is the same concept that Dr. Sperry discovered. Spinal movement charges the brain's 'batteries'. Spinal movement powers your nervous system only if you maintain movement if you are to have a fully powered, nervous system. So, what happens when a joint is unable to move? Until this joint is aligned, to allow motion, the receptors in that joint will not fire at their full potential and the brain and spinal cord won't be fully stimulated. Power shortage! Since you now know that 'life' is responsible for misalignment, you must consistently restore freedom of movement - so how do we do that?

Two Paths to Nervous System Health

You have two opportunities that work hand in hand, to create a vibrant and healthy nervous system:

1. Spinal Maintenance
2. Movement Therapy

1. Spinal Maintenance

Most people don't attend to their spine until they are well into their 20's or 30's and beyond. And it's usually prompted by pain. This may be you, or perhaps you may have never attended to the health of your spine. Well, it's time to begin because you may have already accumulated stress damage responsible for pain, discomfort or nervous system interference. Misalignments and early degeneration of the spine are already present, and your nervous system is already reacting, so it's time to reboot your nervous system, balance your muscles and align your joints. Strive to achieve and maintain optimal movement in your spine: that's where your greatest number of nervous system 'charge-up' receptors are found. Here are 4 Ways to Reboot, Reset and Restore:

#1 **Chiropractic** is gaining popularity in the pain care arena in light of the 'Opioid Crisis' but it goes beyond pain care. Chiropractic focuses on the spine and the nervous system as a primary concern for optimal health. Maintenance of nerve-structural balance is achieved by restoring alignment. Chiropractors specialize in the treatment of structural balance throughout the body, the spine and the effects on the nerves around and inside the spine that communicate with the brain. An example is the vagus nerve which passes through the upper neck and supplies impulses for breathing, blood pressure, bowel movements, immunity, hormone balance, and reproduction. Chiropractors alignments remove interference of the vagus nerve to restore nerve impulses from the brain to the body. When the spine is out of alignment, it irritates and distorts nerve messages causing damage and compromising the body's self-healing processes.

#2 Osteopathy is based on impaired function from a loss of movement. It emphasizes relationships of structure and function, with an appreciation of the body's ability to heal itself. Body systems are united through the nervous, endocrine and circulatory systems. In the study of health and disease, no part of the body is considered autonomous. Originally osteopaths did not use more invasive techniques (medicines, injections, surgery, etc.) however in the USA that unfortunately changed, and their main treatment uses invasive techniques. It is difficult to find osteopaths that practice in the original philosophy but there are a few out there.

#3 Massage involves two main components: touch and pressure. Attaining a balance between the two is an important skill. The most commonly used technique is Swedish massage although many others exist, including deep-tissue, Rolfing, sports massage and acupressure. The main goals of massage are to relieve pain, reduce swelling, relax muscles and support healing. Massage is the manipulation of body tissues, performed primarily with the hands on the nervous, circulatory and muscular systems. Deep massage is used to restore freedom of movement and posture.

#4 Reflexology maps out the reflexes on the feet and hands which connects to all the organs of the body. It involves the application of pressure to the hands or feet to produce effects in other body regions which are divided into different zones. Reflexology suggests a link between organs within these zones and has charted areas in the foot that correspond to areas of the body. Reflexologists do not seek to diagnose medical conditions.

2. Movement Therapy

When you walk, run, stretch, or resist movements, you create a body charge-up equivalent to the watch winding scenario we described earlier. As you exercise, imagine the receptors of your spine lighting up and sending energy to your spinal cord and up to your brain. The more joint movement, the more you illuminate. Sadly, we too often see degeneration in too many people from a lack of movement- it is as if someone has turned down their body's dimmer switch. They are not illuminated, and they function at a very low energy level. This 'dimming down' often includes brain fog, a slow metabolism, weight gain and sleep issues. In the Exercise Chapter, you will learn about our **Structural Reset** exercise program that is customized for anyone at any age. Here are 4 movement therapies to consider:

#1 **Alexander Technique:** encourages you to expend a minimum of effort to achieve the maximum efficient use of your muscles and movement with the aim of relieving pain, improving posture and overall health. The technique involves a process of psychophysical re-education that engages your mind and body. Through the teacher's hands, you focus attention on areas of undue muscle tension. This kinesthetic experience helps release tension and increases understanding how to use postural muscles to support your structure and improve your alignment.

#2 **Feldenkrais Method:** similar to the Alexander technique, it is viewed as an educational system for the development of self-awareness, which relies on your body as the learning instrument. It is designed to help you reorganize and recall forgotten movement patterns.

#3 Yoga: Hatha combines a series of basic postures with breathing. Vinyasa is a series of poses that flow smoothly into one another. Power yoga is a faster, higher-intensity practice. Ashtanga combines poses with breathing techniques. Bikram or 'hot yoga' is a series of 26 poses in a room heated to a high temperature. Iyengar uses props like blocks, straps, and chairs to help support your body alignment.

#4 Pilates: We have used Pilates apparatus in our clinic for years for everything from post-surgical hip replacement therapy to helping professional dancers perform better. It teaches symmetry of movement as joints are worked muscle by muscle, taking into account flexibility, function and stability. Pelvic stability is maintained with abdominal exercises and breathing. All exercises create balance (alignment), improved posture, flexibility and a longer, leaner look for your body.

Case Study #2: John; Osteoarthritis

John was a 54 year old man who was suffering with lower back pain for 10 years, knee pain for 7 years and shoulders pain for two years. He had seen his general physician, a rheumatologist, physical therapist, orthopedist and had an MRI, X-rays and blood tests which found arthritis in his back. Treatment consisted of prescription anti-inflammatory drugs and a variety of natural remedies he tried on his own. This Disease Centered Approach was not helping him, and the medication was causing stomach problems. I evaluated him and immediately started him on an anti-inflammatory lifestyle plan and after 2 weeks, his pain was reduced 50%. I sent him for therapeutic massage and chiropractic adjustments and within 4 weeks his pain was reduced by 80%, and he stopped all arthritis and pain medications under his doctor's supervision. I started him on Pilates exercise to reprogram muscle malfunctions which led to weight training in a gym. In 6 weeks he was 95% better and had all the tools he needed to take care of himself.

Note: We never recommend discontinuing medications without consulting your prescribing doctor.

The Value Of Alignment

Movement Therapies are important for your nervous system and general overall health, but it's critical to keep your spine aligned with corrective care. This is critical for your autonomic nerve pathway described earlier in this chapter, which involves nerves in the brain, the spinal cord that connects to a ganglia (gang of nerves) that connect to your organs.

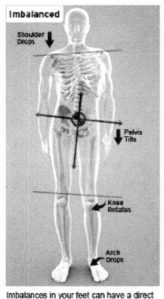

Imbalances in your feet can have a direct effect on your knees, hips, back and neck.

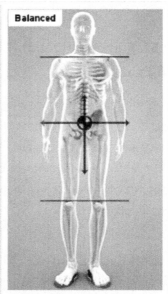

Stabilizing Orthotics can help you have a balanced foundation and can improve your overall health.

How To Determine If Your Structure Is Prematurely Aging

Here are 8 ways to scientifically determine the age and therefore health of your structure:

Tests For Premature Structural Aging
1. Standing Evaluation: Posture
2. Gait Evaluation: Posture and the feet
3. Muscle Tone Evaluation
4. Strength Test: Movements and timing of individual muscle groups
5. Flexibility / Range of motion
6. Muscle Mass
7. X-rays and MRI
8. Bone Density

Test 1: Standing Evaluation—Posture and Central Nervous System Examination

Perhaps the most important thing you can learn from an observation of posture is that you understand the importance of examining, measuring and quantifying all that can be known about posture changes. Muscles keep joints in center, but you must have proper alignment first in order to reset your posture for optimal function and damage protection.

Test 2: Gait Evaluation

You can actually stop pain by changing the way you walk, run and stand. Orthotic correction (custom inserts for your shoes) of supination of the foot and ankle and external rotation of the leg stabilizes your pelvis and provides a more horizontal foundation for the entire spine.

We have seen over and over that orthotics can reverse years of poor posture and help runners, cyclists, and many other athletes to enhance performance. Orthotics often help you avoid foot surgery.

Test 3: Muscle Tone

Electromyograph (EMG) measures muscle activity at rest. Constant irritation of the spine causes cells to become exhausted and die. This is reversible if you start with the right approach. EMG can be a good way to test the health of your muscles.

Hands on Assessment is a great test for muscle spasms, knots or trigger points to help determine if you have tight or overactive muscles.

Test 4: Strength

A Dynamometer measures strength or force. There is equipment that tests all the muscles in the body and it is a great way to measure progress.

Test 5: Flexibility

Goniometers measure any restrictions you may have with your range or motion for different areas of your body.

Test 6: Muscle Mass

Underwater testing is the most accurate test of muscle mass, but not practical. A quality Bioelectric Impedance Analysis (BIA) is more practical and accurate, but beware of poor quality units or standing devices that only measure the lower half of your body.

Test 7: MRI and X-rays

"'Let's get an MRI to see if there is anything wrong with the spine' is the beginning of a dangerous thought process."

~ Renowned spine scientist Dr. Scott Boden MD.

Studies show that patients who get MRI's have WORSE outcomes than patients who do not. The majority of people with back pain have problems with poor muscle flexibility, strength, or endurance and none of this shows up on an MRI. There is no proof that abnormalities found on MRIs (disc tears, bulges, herniation, or degeneration) cause pain. A study in the New England Journal of Medicine found that the majority, 64 percent of people without any pain, have disc tears, bulges and herniations! The authors of the study concluded that disc bulges are a normal part of aging in both men and women.

In some cases, doctors use MRI's and X-rays to justify treatment and surgery. You hear the phrase "Bone on bone" and its straight to the operating room! The fact is, you can have a beautiful MRI or X-ray, and still be in massive pain. You can also have an MRI that looks like a Nightmare on Elm Street and have very little pain or no pain whatsoever! We're not saying these tests are meaningless, but too often they are given far too much weight in our decisions.

Another study found that only 1 out of 2,500 X-rays of the spine showed anything helpful in determining an individual's back pain. So, when I look at an MRI or X-Ray film and see a film of a 40-year-old that looks like it belongs to an 80-year-old, it can be disturbing-however, what we see on a film does not always dictate your care.

Test 8: Bone Mass Density Test

The DEXA scan measures the strength of your bones. The main reason to have the test is to find osteoporosis and prevent fractures. Most people under age 65 don't need the test because they don't have serious bone loss. They just have osteopenia and their risk of fracture is very low and since the test gives off radiation, it is best to avoid it if you can until you are over 65.

Actions Steps:

REBOOT! How Much Time Is Needed To Correct Imbalances In Your Posture?

Everybody is unique. Most of us have had abnormal posture for years and sometimes decades. So how long does it take to reset, reboot and correct posture?

Just like an orthodontist correcting the teeth with braces, it takes time to correct posture. Research shows the minimum length of time is 9 weeks, however, it may take 6 months to 1 year for full correction. You may need to continue your exercises until restored, or if you continue to subject yourself to repetitive stress injury from poor ergonomic conditions. Stay consistent until you reach maximum improvement or that you have reached an optimal amount of correction.

But understand, it's not the total time spent exercising . . . *it's the biological response it creates.* That's where the magic is found. You are learning to manage 95% of your body's needs for health. Just as you are ultimately responsible for taking care of all other aspects of your health—the same holds true for alignment of your spine and nervous system. Combine periodic, corrective alignments to your spine and joints with the movement therapy described in this chapter; you can't help but power your system up, light your system up and ensure the best opportunity you have toward an abundant and fulfilling life.

Actions steps

1. **Find a reputable spinal maintenance team:** You don't have to be hurting to get a check-up. In truth, if you wait until you're hurting, your recovery will be much slower, and some damage is less likely to be reversible.
2. **Get moving:** Exercise intelligently and efficiently!

TOTAL NUTRITION

Regimen
Educational Curriculum
Coaching
Reducing Inflammation
Endocrine System
Alignment of Your Structure
Total Nutrition
Exercise

"Health Gain = Weight Loss"

~ Judy Pearson Kobsar

STOP <u>TRYING</u> TO LOSE WEIGHT! A meal plan focused on your health will burn the fat away permanently not just temporarily.

"The biggest Health discovery of the past 30 years is that food isn't just energy. It literally provides instructions on a bite-by-bite basis to every chemical reaction in your body. In fact, you change your gene expression with every bite. You change your metabolic age, either for good or the bad, when you change your relationship to food. There's no drugs that can heal like food does. Crippling, chronic disease can be pain-free in weeks and you can get off expensive drugs. Food truly is medicine and when you realize that you can transform your health".

~ Dr. Mark Hyman

The Macmillan Dictionary states that the definition of food is "that which is eaten to sustain life, provide energy, and promote growth and repair of tissues." The average 'American high glycemic load diet' does <u>not</u> fit that description. The average American diet provides short term energy causing unstable blood sugar, hormone imbalance, weight gain and disease. Optimal health must include a good nutrients and food for your cells- this will always be what brings about health and weight loss. The good news is that it doesn't have to be bland. Good, whole food nutrition is full of flavor and exciting recipes that burst with deliciousness!

What The Heck Is A Balanced Diet?!

You may often hear if you just eat a balanced diet everything will magically fall into place, yet 80% of Americans dont eat a balanced diet. Well, just what is this mythical balanced diet that we hear so much about? The truth is, there isn't one. The problem is that a balanced diet is different for everyone because we are all genetically, metabolically, hormonally, unique. We have different body types, different genders, different height and weight and so forth. Since we are all unique it only makes sense that our diet should be unique as well. A balanced diet provides the building block for all body functions, in t*he right amount, at the right time.*

Large-scale deficiencies of nutrients in our population are well documented in extensive government-sponsored research and a tsunami of scientific evidence shows that nutrients are essential for a healthy metabolism. We use the word Total when we discuss Nutrition because after years of looking at lab tests, we've seen a rising tide in the number of people that are malnourished. And this includes the people that eat only organic foods from the farmers markets or health food grocery stores. How can this be? We've found two reasons:

1. **The food industry has worked relentlessly to increase profits by replacing real food (short shelf life) with fake food that lasts forever on grocery store shelves.** They fill our food with cheap preservatives and toxic additives and then lobby for laws that allow them to hide it on the food labels.

2. **Our soil is depleted.** Before big corporations took over, farmers rotated their crops every year. They only planted crops every other year, so the soil could replenish the nutrients. That practice is long gone along with most 'mom and pop' farms. Big corporations own most of the farming but their marketing is often made to disguise themselves at local farmers markets in their 'mom and pop farmer disguise' so the public is fooled into believing they are supporting family farm produce.

We are saddened by how many people make poor health choices based on their trust in their government and the food industry. But the loudest voices that are leading our country (and still are) in a rapid downward health spiral are the processed food and fast-food industries. This mirrors how the pharmaceutical companies have infiltrated our medical system and Coke, Pepsi Co and others have infiltrated our schools. Those voices tell us in their endless advertising and world-class marketing lingo that they "bring good things to life." They want to influence your thoughts with their **big, FAT lies.** The processed food industry is the only one who benefits because cheap, calorie-loaded, trans-fat, chemically addictive products are so very profitable. The junk is everywhere and it's making our country, and more than likely YOU, sick! These 10 Food Conglomerates control 90% of the food supply:

- Kellogg's
- Mars
- General Mills
- Johnson and Johnson
- Wrigley's
- Kraft
- PepsiCo
- Coca Cola
- Nestles
- Unilever

These companies have worked very hard to convince us that food is just calories. The fact is, food is information, and the American high-glycemic diet is telling your genes to express diabetes and obesity-to turn on those genes. Obesity steals nine years of life from the average person as reported in the March 2016 journal, the *Lancet*. Obesity in adolescents has the same risk of early death as heavy smoking reported in the March 2009 *British Medical Journal*. Diabetes and obesity are not genetic disorders in the strictest sense. While it's true that your inherited genes may put you at greater risk, it doesn't mean you must get diabetes or become obese. These conditions are a direct outcome of lifestyle, and environmental factors turning on the wrong genes.

The great news is if your genes can be switched on, they can be switched off. If you are over-weight, sick, stressed and tired, it's time to at least consider a different approach—something suited to your specific metabolic and hormonal needs. A program based on the latest science and most importantly, a program you can **stick** with. A program that does not focus solely on weight loss but on restoring and staying healthy. A program that makes a '**MIND SHIFT**' in your lifestyle '**MINDSET**' like many of our Wellness Partners have experienced. They came to us sick, medicated, and frustrated with the avalanche of weight loss programs, diet plans, diet pills, that claim to help you get that summer bathing suit body. Studies show that 95% of people who go on the big name brand diets fail. And often, they end up heavier than they were when they started. Nearly all the diet books on the best-seller lists neglect to tell you that if you follow their instructions and make a temporary change in your eating habits, your weight loss will most likely also become **temporary.** It's high time to understand that food is not just calories, it is information sending messages to your body to store fat or burn fat. When you learn that, you learn to eat to recover your health and fat loss is side effect of this.

Macronutrient And Micronutrients:

A Balanced Diet must combine these in the right amount, at the right time.

Macronutrients consist of:

- Carbohydrates- Immediate energy. Only energy source for the brain.
- Proteins -Intermediate energy. Building and repair of organs, muscles, and enzymes.
- Fats - Long term energy. Building cell membranes, steroid hormones and nerve conduction.

Micronutrients consist of:

- Vitamins and Minerals - energy, immune function, control blood sugar and reduce inflammation.
- Amino Acids - needed for enzymes and proteins to function properly.
- Fatty Acids and Anti-oxidants—neutralize free radicals and support hormones.

TOTAL NUTRITION combines all the nutrients you require from the two major categories of nutrients: MACROnutrients and MICROnutrients. Both are equally important to your vital health, though you hear more about macronutrients since that is how you choose the food you eat every day for your energy source. (low carb, high fat, etc.) Micronutrients give you the raw materials and building blocks you need for all your cellular system and body functions. Macronutrients provides you the energy needed to maintain body functions and carry out the daily activities of life. An easy way to differentiate between the two is to think of your MICROnutrients as the 'small picture' of your diet while your MACROnutrients are the 'big picture.' Both are essential to maintaining your hormone balance and sustaining a youthful metabolism for optimal health. However, they only work if you are eating quality whole foods and whole food supplements in the right amounts and the correct dose. Do this and they will be all the medicine you will ever need to keep all the systems of your body running at maximum capacity.

A major function of micronutrients is to break down your macronutrients (food) so that you can use their energy. You may be less familiar with MICROnutrients, but this doesn't make them any less important. Many micronutrients are 'essential nutrients', which means they can't be made by your body. We must get these micronutrients from foods, in the right balance, or we get sick and diseases like anemia (iron, B12 or B6 imbalance), high blood pressure, heart arrhythmia, muscle pain and cramping (magnesium, calcium imbalance) and even sudden death (potassium, sodium imbalance). Scientists have classified 13 different types of vitamins, all of which are important in protecting you from inflammation, slowing your aging process and preventing cancer. But we are getting ahead of ourselves so let's go back and fill in the blanks on the big picture 'macronutrients' first.

Macronutrients And Metabolism

Macronutrients are chemically different from micronutrients and have a different function and hormone response. This means the kind of calories you consume have a big impact on weight gain, because different types of food are metabolized in different ways. Protein helps produce hormones that build muscle, the more muscle you have the more calories you burn 24 hours a day, 7 days a week. After eating carbohydrates, the body increases insulin to move sugars and protein into the cells, storing any extra sugar as fat. Eating fat has little immediate influence on hormone balance however hormones are made from fat, so it does have an influence over time.

Why The Most Popular Weight Loss Plans Fail In The Long Run

You've got to recognize that being overweight is nothing more than poor health. The ultimate goal is to improve the efficiency of your metabolism and balance your hormones. As this happens, you will not only get healthier, but you will steadily drop fat and increase lean muscle mass until you finally reach your ideal body weight. You may be asking if our Wellness Method Program will help you lose 10 pounds in the first week or will it help you lose 20 pounds in the first month. Well our answer is maybe, but it depends on where your health is at. Because, once we understand the cause of your weight gain and learn exactly what you need to do to lose fat, your weight loss will be permanent!

BIG FAT LIE: To Lose Weight, Just Cut Calories. All Calories Are Created Equal.

Fact: If you have a stubborn weight problem, the last thing you should do is cut calories because it doesn't work. IT DOESN'T WORK! By the way, did we say *IT DOESN'T WORK?* We understand the habitual beliefs that have pervaded our society for years and years, therefore our voice must be louder and more constant in order to wake you up!

Here's why it doesn't work: The truth is there are good calories and there are bad calories. Metabolism is more than a simple math problem. When you eat, your food interacts with your physiology which is a complex adaptive system that transforms with every bite. Every bite affects your hormones, your brain chemistry and your metabolism. You see, sugar calories cause fat storage and they spike your blood sugar and that slows your metabolism. Whereas, protein and fat calories promote more fat burning. What counts even more than calories is the quality of those calories.

Remember when we talked about Inflammation in a previous chapter? Everyone is inflamed and that causes your metabolism to run slow. After reducing inflammation, the next step for many is to fix your metabolism. When you do this, you don't have to count calories and you'll lose fat that stays off for good. The idea that 'as long as we burn more calories than we eat we'll lose weight' is simply wrong and outdated. 'Just eat less and exercise more' is a mantra you hear from the food industry, from our government agencies and from too many doctors and dietitians. This message unfortunately is not driven with your best interest in mind. The science is clear, and our experience with our thousands of Wellness Partners is irrefutable. Food is information for your cells and systems of your body, therefore it needs to be treated with the respect that it deserves. If you can do that, your health will dramatically change, and so will your life.

Calorie Counting – A Futile Endeavor

Many factors besides calories affect your weight, so if you fail to consider the other important factors, calorie counting will fail. Counting as a way of keeping weight down does not work because counting calories is not the same as burning them. There are so many factors that modify the rate at which your body burns calories that simply regulating the number of calories you consume is ineffective in the battle against the bulge. The calorie values of foods printed on labels and in diet books assume that foods containing them are completely burned or oxidized. In reality, your body burns some foods better than others, and there are individual differences in food burning ability.

What Are Good-Quality Calories? A simpler approach and more effective approach that makes calorie tables and charts unnecessary is called "Whole Foods". Eating whole foods - fresh food like your great grandmother made- all organic but we never had to call it that because genetically modified food did not exist yet. Good quality protein, grass fed animal products not factory farmed. Organic eggs, chicken, small wild fish, nuts and seeds, good carbs. Ok, let's get clear on carbs for a minute- we love carbs, in fact most of our diet is carbs! But we eat vibrantly colored, non-starchy vegetables which are 'fibrous carbs', not starchy-carbs. The brighter the color the better, and you can binge on these as much as you want! Have 5 pounds of bell peppers if you want, go crazy . . . and have good fruits that are low sugar like berries and apples and kiwi's and watermelon to your heart's content! And include super foods like chia and hemp seeds along with lots of good fats like avocados, extra-virgin olive oil, all kinds of nuts and seeds, coconut oil, butter and omega-3 fats from fish. Consuming these types of foods on a regular basis will free you from calorie counting and free you from your fat stores!

Your Metabolism Is Too Slow And Too Old

We hear people talk about metabolism all the time, but it's really very simple- if your metabolism is older than you are and slower than you are, then your inflammation is too high, and your hormones are out of whack! These two issues must get repaired first and foremost before real, sustainable weight loss will occur. Being overweight almost never is primarily associated with over eating. In fact, most people who are overweight are mal-nourished because their stomach stopped working and they are not getting the proper nutrients. That, in fact, is one of the main reasons why a large percentage of people are overweight—because— their body goes into a defensive state thinking it is suffering from starvation because it is so poorly nourished. Under these conditions, your body wants to grab every bit of food that is taken in and store it as fat as a defensive measure- in case you never eat again. Also, the body tends to slow its metabolism down as a defensive measure to conserve energy (calories)- again, in case you never get to eat again. The slower the metabolism gets, the more and more difficult it becomes to lose weight. Your body is protecting itself from what it believes is starvation.

Metabolic Rate

Metabolic rates differ from one person to another because your genes, hormones, nutrition, exercise all affect your metabolic rate and your overall state of health. Your friend or spouse may have a high metabolic rate and never gain weight while you eat very little and can't seem to lose any weight, which, come on! HOW IS THAT FAIR?! Well, aside from hating on these people what can you do about this?

Metabolic Age

The key to losing weight and keeping it off is to simply improve your calorie burning capabilities- and that is the 'mind set' you must shift into. Restoring your metabolism and lowering your 'metabolic age' turns you into a fat burning machine instead of a fat storing, calorie counting machine. You will learn sound scientific practices to improve your metabolic function in these next chapters. Hear us on this- your body will fight you all the way if all you do is drastically reduce the calories you take in, it just will not work. The best method to keeping body fat down is an effective metabolism and functioning hormones. The secret to starting and keeping the metabolic-fire burning will be **FOOD**, yes food and a lot more than you are used to. You will actually be able to eat and lose weight. Food will become your friend. Your new motto will be, "Eat More to Lose More".

Let's begin with small effective changes in your habits. Good food and the right kind of exercise are essential, but you have to start with restoring your health! This is where the endless stream of fad, weight loss diets that come and go fall short completely. They do nothing to restore your health, and often make your health worse! The research shows when you go off those diets, all your weight and more comes back with a vengeance . . . so now we want to share how to lower your Metabolic Age. Let's start with the macronutrients—Protein, Carbs and Fats:

Protein

Protein is made up of amino acids which are necessary for many bodily functions including making muscle. If there aren't enough amino acids from your diet, your body will make them from wherever it can grab them- and muscle is the richest source. This 'protein steal' means, you are losing muscle, and lowering your metabolism. You will not be able to increase calorie burning muscle if you're not taking in enough protein. Here's how to make protein work for you:

Step 1: Add a protein source to every meal and snack

This will ramp up your metabolism and ensure a steady supply of amino acids are present for muscle building and other needed processes of the body. Eating protein increases metabolism by 14%, so that alone is a good reason to include protein with every meal and snack.

Step 2: How Much Protein?

Figuring out your protein needs is not a straight-forward equation. There are some things to consider:

1. How active are you? If you are not very active you will need less protein than someone who is active.

2. Are you recovering from injury or surgery? This will increase your demand for protein which is needed for repair of tissues.

3. As your need for protein increases, your need for carbs and fat increases, so there is an optimal ratio that must be attained.

* Beware of the notion that 'increasing protein and reducing carbs will make you leaner.' Your body will respond by breaking down muscle to make sugar in the body. This will slow your metabolism, reduce your testosterone by 15-20 % and increase Cortisol.

Protein and Carbohydrate Formula

Protein: Divide your body weight by 15.

Example: A 180-pound man divided by 15 = 12 ounces of protein (meat, fish, eggs, poultry). If you divide by three meals, the result is about 4 ounces of protein per meal.

Carbohydrate: Multiply the ounces of protein above per day x 10 to get carbohydrate needs. A little higher for the underweight and a little lower for the overweight person.

Example: 180-pound man multiplies 10 x 12 = 120 ounces carbs/day. This breaks down to about 40 ounces carbs /meal.

Protein Builds Muscle, And Muscle Burns Fat

It is the **energy demands** of building muscle, **not the need for protein,** that needs consideration. High protein diets do not equal weight loss. The question is, how much protein can you assimilate from one meal? A consideration as to upper limits of protein intake is related to how quickly amino acids (protein is made of amino acids) get transported to blood and how quickly they then get assimilated into muscle. Here are a few proteins and their absorption rates to give you an idea of how this works:

- Egg protein absorbed at 1. 3 grams/hour
- Casein isolate (a protein found in dairy) absorbed at 6. 1 grams/hour
- Whey isolate absorbed at 8-10 grams/hour

If an average protein absorption rate of about 7 grams/hour can be estimated by this research, then the upper limit of absorption is approximately 168 grams /day. (24 hours x 7). If this is accurate, the **high protein diets don't make sense.** So, can problems arise from eating too much protein? **Absolutely.** As stated earlier, high protein, to low carbohydrate ratio can lead to muscle breakdown to supply sugar to the body and lowers your anabolic capacity. The above formula ensures sufficient protein and carbohydrate intake for optimal health and fitness.

Protein Shakes

We encourage the use of a high-quality, hypoallergenic rice, pea, hemp or chia protein powder. Some of these powders are anti-inflammatory and support detoxification. A protein shake also makes an excellent breakfast and snack option, helping balance your blood sugar and heal your liver.

Carbohydrates

Have you ever skipped a meal and then felt that ravenous hunger where all you want is carbs? Then you binge and feel like you've satisfied your hunger? Well, if you've done that you need to know what you really did was give yourself a huge insulin spike leading to insulin resistance and acidosis and gave yourself zero nutrients that your body can actually use. Insulin spikes cause storage of electrolytes (potassium, magnesium, phosphate) and a drop-in blood potassium and magnesium linked to heart attacks. The rhythm of the heart depends on this balance of intracellular & extracellular electrolytes. So, we want you to know how important it is to eat the right kind of carbs at the right times.

Sugar

Sugar is a simple carbohydrate that is rapidly absorbed in your body- honey, table sugar, candy, deserts, sodas, etc. . Sugar causes accelerated aging and chronic disease, so we want to provide a guide to understanding this type of carbohydrate consumption.

- **0 to 50 grams per day** - Not practical as a long - term practice but will accelerate weight loss under Doctor Supervision.
- **50-100 grams per day**- The 'sweet spot' for optimal health to accelerate fat metabolism
- **100 to 150 grams per day**- Used to maintain weight.
- **150 to 300 grams per day**- Contributes to widespread sickness.
- **300 or more grams per day-** For the non-athlete this is the "Danger Zone"and the primary catalyst for chronic disease.

*As you include intense exercise, these numbers can be adjusted up slightly along with protein and fat.

"If sugar were just empty calories, then we wouldn't have seen a worsening of the problems, but we did, and the reason is because sugar is not just empty calories. Sugar[s] are toxic calories because of the way fructose is metabolized in the liver. Non-alcoholic fatty liver disease wasn't even a disease until 1980, and now it affects 35% of all Americans." Robert Lustig, MD, PhD

BIG FAT LIE: Breakfast Is The Most Important Meal Of The Day.

Make breakfast your largest meal and dinner your smallest meal. You may have been told this but for most people it's just not true.

Fact: The reality is, not everyone needs breakfast. Our high glycemic American diet has made so many people solely dependent on sugar for energy. This causes your blood sugar to be so unstable that if you go more than a couple hours without food you can't function. This also can cause you to become insulin resistant and/or leptin resistant. But you can train your body to use your fat cells for energy and to burn ketones instead. This process is called ketogenesis- and intermittent fasting is the best way to break this cycle of sugar dependence and to train our body to start using fat for energy. Skipping breakfast will also help interrupt both of these hormone imbalances. Other hormone imbalances like estrogen, testosterone and cortisol can also create this sugar dependence so it's important to get everything checked out before making changes so you don't set yourself up to fail. Contrary to what you've been told, a healthy lifestyle is not painful or time consuming. Simple changes like this one produce gigantic improvements in your health—and the only way to lose fat and keep it off permanently is to restore your health. Skipping breakfast isn't right for everyone, so it's important to be under guidance of a qualified expert in Functional Medicine.

Mainstream media influences your daily lives and unfortunately much of the information you get is biased by those feeding it to you. The primary motivation for companies to disseminate the information they do is their bottom-line profit. This information is not always in **your** best interest. Some of the information we present in this book will surely **contradict** what you have read and been told, but we assure you there is science, research and plenty of clinical experience to back it up.

Danger! HFCS

One sugar that may be worse than any other sweetener is **high-fructose corn syrup (HFCS).** When the processed food industry first introduced HFCS onto the market we were told it was healthy. Now let us explain how the food industry scientists deceived us as consumers: Testing showed that if you consumed HFCS, your blood showed a sugar spike, but it was actually a lower spike than glucose causes. They wanted you to focus on that point . . . and believe that HFCS was not harmful. What they failed to reveal was the fructose (sugar in HFCS) has to get metabolized in the liver BEFORE it reaches the blood stream. So, it takes fructose longer to show a sugar spike . . . and you guessed it, they performed the blood test BEFORE fructose made its way to the blood stream. If they would've waited for the fructose to enter your blood, and then test you, it would show that HFCS spiked your blood sugar TWICE as much as glucose does. Dangerously high! Also, your brain does not recognize HFCS as any kind of real food, so it sends the signal that the body needs to keep eating. Please avoid anything with HFCS in it.

Fiber

Eating high fiber foods creates a sense of fullness after eating. Fiber or roughage is a powerful substance that can absorb fat and sugar in your stomach and lower insulin levels. Fiber slows the transit of food through the digestive system keeping your stomach full longer. An example is eating an apple versus drinking apple juice: they both supply the same nutrients and sugar, but the apple in its whole form requires much more energy and time to digest and the apple has a lower glycemic score due to the fiber. A high fiber diet will lower the 'glycemic load' of your meal by slowing the rate that sugar is digested. You must use real fiber from whole foods not fake fiber found in medications or processed foods. Good sources of fiber include oatmeal, beans, whole grains, vegetables and fruit.

Fats

Omega-6's and Omega-3's

It's important to have the right ratio of these two types of omega fats. When they get unfavorably imbalanced you will see fat redistribution in your gut. The ratio should be 1 to 1, omega 6's to omega 3's but Americans have 20-50x more Omega 6 fats from french fries, processed foods, etc.

Fatty Liver: Organ fat, especially fatty liver is far more common now than it used to be. What used to be an alcoholic liver is now more commonly caused by high fructose as reported by Robert Lustig MD, PhD out of University of California San Francisco. We now have non-alcoholic fatty liver. This tells you why eliminating good fats is causing you to store more fat. By eliminating them you are eating more **refined and processed foods with sugar.** By adding good protein sources with some fat and fiber from fruits and vegetables, you keep your blood sugar constant which means *Less Fat Stored!*

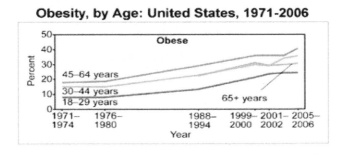

Obesity, by Age: United States, 1971-2006

BIG FAT LIE: Saturated Fat causes disease according to the government ... Wrong!

Fact: If saturated fats really cause disease, none of us would be here because saturated fat was the primary energy source of our ancestors. Additionally, the World War II generation feasted on breakfasts of steak and eggs and yet obesity was very RARE, showing in only 10% of the population, and diabetes was very uncommon. But this was all about to change ... beginning in the 1960's animal fat in the American diet declined from 83% to 62%. Butter consumption dropped from 18 lbs. per person per year to only 4 lbs. per person per year. Over the past 50 years, vegetable oils in the form of margarine, shortening and refined oils increased 400%!! And since the 1970's when the American Heart Association implemented their low-fat diet advice obesity has tripled. Sugar and trans fats are killing us, they are toxic to the body, not saturated fats.

Good Fats—Bad Fats

Processed foods are laden with trans-fatty acids (TFAs) which are closer to plastic in molecular structure than fat. Ever wonder how that box of crackers could have an expiration date of a few years from now? Try leaving real food out for that long! Chemists learned that exposing cooking oils to temperatures over 400 degrees fahrenheit and adding hydrogen to it will keep these oils from going rancid even without refrigeration. This chemical processing of oils at high temperatures changes the molecule into a shape that damages the human body and your ability to metabolize cholesterol, therefore causing high cholesterol. We have known about this for years, but the warnings of Harvard researchers have been continually ignored. TFA consumption is linked to heart disease, cancer, creates weight gain, etc. Doctors instruct patients with high LDL's to restrict butter, cheese, eggs, red meat and eat a low-fat diet high in grains and vegetables and margarine. All of which is making the problem worse! Margarine is notorious for high TFAs along with crackers, snack foods, frozen dinners, bread, cereals and the oil used in deep-frying. Avoid foods that list "hydrogenated" or "partially hydrogenated" vegetable shortening or vegetable oil among the ingredients.

Bad Fats	**Saturated Fats:** Sources: animal products, coconut and palm oil
• Trans-fats, Hydrogenated or partially hydrogenated	• Needed for proper use of Essential Fatty Acids
• Oils (corn, safflower, soy and cottonseed)	• Enhance immune system
Good Fats	• Needed for calcium to be effectively used by the bones
• Olive oil, Coconut Oil, Macadamia Oil, Palm Oil	• Main component of cell membranes
• Butter, Flax seeds, Avocados, Nuts (raw, organic)	**Monosaturated Fats** Sources: olive oil, almonds, cashews, peanuts, avocados
• Organic, grass fed animal fats	• Liquid at room temperature
• Fish oil (be careful of sources)	• Can be used in cooking at moderate temperatures

BIG FAT LIE: Cholesterol is evil. Lie! This lie has possibly kept you from enjoying foods that are good for your metabolism.
Fact: The truth is, your liver produces about 2000 milligrams of cholesterol every day! Do you think your body is trying to kill you? Of course not. Your brain, hormones and every cell in your body is made up of cholesterol. Only when cholesterol is 'oxidized' does it become a problem. Do you know what happens if you follow the low cholesterol diet? Your cholesterol goes up! The reason this happens is that your liver produces more cholesterol to ensure you have enough. In fact, we've known for more than 5 years that high cholesterol in your blood is not even a primary risk factor

for heart attacks and strokes. For decades it was assumed that because high cholesterol accompanies cardiovascular disease it was the CAUSE of heart attacks and strokes. But studies have reported people with low cholesterol are three times as likely to have a stroke than the average person. And as far as heart attacks go, more people who have fatal heart attacks actually have LOW cholesterol! That's right, you can eat eggs! Unadulterated eggs are, in fact, not only an excellent source of protein; they're also a great source of dietary fats.

**Note: If you eat a lot of eggs you need to buy free-range eggs as opposed to conventionally raised eggs because of the imbalance of omega 3 to omega 6 which causes inflammation. Look for a dark orange yolk as opposed to light yellow.

A study published in the Journal of the American Medical Association, 1999; 281 (15); 1387-94) showed no connection between eating eggs and the risk of heart disease or stroke. In another study on exercise and fat intake by Leddy published in 1997 in Medicine and Science in Sports and Exercise, elite endurance athletes were put on a high fat diet first and then a low-fat diet. On the high saturated fat diet, the athletes maintained low body fat, weight and triglycerides. When put on a low fat, high carb diet they had a major drop in HDL (good) cholesterol, increased triglycerides and increased the ratio of triglyceride to HDL ratio which is a risk factors for cardiovascular disease. One more study- The Journal of Lipid Research, 2000; 4 1 (5): 834-39), showed that eating vegetable oils in the form of either soy or margarine raised LDL (bad cholesterol) and lowered HDL (good cholesterol). But eating butter lowered LDL cholesterol and raised HDL cholesterol.

Coconut Oil: "Good" Fat

Coconut oil contains a fat called lauric acid which experts consider a "miracle" ingredient because it's converted by the body into monolaurin, which has anti-viral, anti-bacterial properties that actually destroy viruses such as herpes, measles, flu virus, and more! It also contains medium chain triglycerides (MCTs). Researchers found that weight loss associated with coconut oil is related to the length of fatty acid chains. Vegetable oils like sunflower, corn, soy, safflower, canola, cotton seed contain long chain triglycerides (LCT's) which get stored in fat cells, while MCTs burn up quickly for energy. In a study at the School of Dietetics and Nutrition, McGill University, 24 overweight men consumed diets high in MCT or LCT for 28 days. "Consumption of a diet rich in MCTs had more loss of body fat compared with LCTs".

Let's review:

To get your fire burning so your fat simply melts off, you need to ramp up your metabolism and become metabolically younger. We've also established some myths and lies that we want to recap. If you want a robust metabolism:

- It is not low-calorie diets.
- It is not diet pills.
- It is not excess cardio/aerobic exercise.
- It is not fat blockers.
- It is not 95% of what you have read prior to our book.
- It will be all the steps we've given you here that will unlock your fat burning ability.

Let's continue on.

BIG FAT LIE: Eating fat makes you fat. Lie! It's the inability to burn fat that makes you fat. Overweight people burn carbs easily, but not fat stores. It takes the right method to become a fat burner and fat is critical to health.

Fact: Fat is not a four-letter word. Studies comparing identical high calorie fat diets compared to high calorie sugar diets have totally different effects on your metabolism. Higher fat diets cause you to burn an extra 300 calories/day compared to a high sugar diet. So, let's take two groups that eat a 1600 calorie/day diet. The group that eats a 60% fat diet burns 300 more calories/day than the group that eats a 60% carbohydrates/day. That is like running an hour a day. This alone would solve the obesity epidemic! Fat speeds up your metabolism while sugar slows it down. Another study in animals found that a high fat, high protein diet not only burned more calories compared to a high sugar, high protein diet, but subjects also gained more muscle mass. Be sure to stay away from the trans fats and vegetable oil fats. Fat is essential for many bodily functions- if it is the good fat! Of course, having too much of this good stuff, as with anything, leads to being overweight and lack of energy.

Micronutrients Vitamin And Minerals, The Co-Factors In Fat Metabolism

BIG FAT LIE: I can get all the nutrients I need from food. Registered dieticians and other health professionals in the standard health care model have sold us for decades on this, even in the face of all contrary research and science in their own science journals! They still repeat the mantra they are taught in school. "You can get all nutrients from the diet we give you." On the surface, it may seem possible. After all, if you eat whole, fresh, unprocessed foods, shouldn't you be able to get all your vitamins, minerals, antioxidants, essential fats, etc.?

FACT: 70 Diets were computer analyzed from the menu of people striving for a toxic free, high quality, micronutrient rich diet and food choices to actively improve nutritional intake. **RESULTS:** Not a single diet achieved the minimum micronutrient suggested by the American Dietic Association. Journal International Sports Nutrition. 2006

Additionally, Fairfield reported in the Journal of the American Medical Association in 2002, that even with a perfect diet, the combination of many factors—our depleted soils, the storage and transportation of food, genetic changes to food, increased stress of modern living and our toxic environment—make it impossible for us to get all the vitamins and minerals we need solely from food. Simply put, the evidence shows we cannot get away from the need for nutritional supplements.

Essential Nutrients: These can't be made by the body. We need these micronutrients, in the right balance, or we risk sickness and disease:

Sickness and Diseases	Needed Vitamins, Minerals, Anti-Oxidants, Enzymes
Inflammatory and Autoimmune Disease: Diabetes, Cancer, Heart Disease, Arthritis, Obesity, Alzheimer's, Parkinson's,	Scientists have classified 13 different vitamins which are important in protecting you from disease, slowing your aging process and preventing cancer. Some of these include vitamin A, Beta-carotene, vitamin E, etc. . . .
Anemia	- B12, B6, or Iron imbalance
- High Blood Pressure - Heart Arrhythmia - Muscle Pain	-Magnesium and Calcium imbalance.
Sudden death	- Potassium and Sodium imbalance.

Supplements are an inexpensive insurance policy to get a full spectrum of all your essential nutrients. **Despite knowing how important supplements are, we did not prescribe supplements for many years for these reasons:**

1. **Fat soluble vitamins and minerals can be toxic.** Excess amounts can't be eliminated so if you don't need them, they create toxicity and inflammation in your cells.
2. **Water soluble vitamins and minerals stress your kidneys and liver.** Excess amounts can be eliminated but you end up putting more unnecessary stress on your organs with the added bonus of literally flushing your money down the toilet.
3. **90% of people we test have a broken digestive system.** You can eat from the Garden of Eden and take bottles of supplements, but if the nutrients aren't absorbed, they are just passing through and you will lack the building blocks needed to rebuild and repair our body every night while you sleep.
4. **Loosely Regulated.** Over-the-counter supplements have no controls placed on them to ensure what is actually in them. Manufacturers often cut corners and distributors like Costco, GNC and Walmart are being sued by the New York Attorney General for selling supplements that do not contain what their label states. This is a problem for you because these supplements:

   - Are cheap, poorly absorbed or not useable by the body.
   - The dosage on the label does not match the dose in the bottle. Only 21% of supplements contained what the label promised according to Consumer Affairs report, 2017.
   - They are filled with additives, colors, fillers, and allergens.
   - 134 products tested and all of them contained at least one heavy metal (Mercury, Arsenic, Lead, Cadmium and all of them contained BPA in their products. Consumer Reports Study 2010 and again in 2018.

Supplements were not personalized for you. There is a lot that needs to be considered for each individual with the right amount of nutrients at the right time. Here are a list of things that need to be considered when prescribing nutritional supplements:

a. BODY TYPE: - Fat, Carbohydrate or Protein burner.

b. GENETICS: - Risks for diabetes, alzheimers, heart disease, cancer, stroke, dimentia, etc . . .

c. METABOLISM: - High, medium or slow.

d. GENDER: - Male / Female

e. AGE: - Child, Adolescent, Adult or Senior.

f. ACTIVITY LEVEL: - Sedentary, low activity, medium activity, high activity, elite athlete.

g. HEALTH: - recovering from physical trauma, Surgery, Disease, Burns, Arthritis, etc . . .

h. MEDICATIONS. - vitamin and mineral deficiencies, main reason for side effects.

i. DIET: - Vegetarian, Paleo, Ketogenic, Low carb, etc . . .

j. PREGNANT/NURSING: - Nutrients for two.

k. SEASONS: - Some seasons require higher doses. ie: Vitamin D in winter.

l. ENVIRONMENT: - Heavy metals, air pollution, water, home cleaning products, skin care, etc.

m. DIGESTION:	- Enzymes; cellulase for starch, lipase for fatty acids, proteolytic for proteins, etc
n. LIFESTYLE:	- Caffeine, alcohol, smoking, exercise, laxatives, stress, sunlight (too much, too little)

We'll explain a little later how we came to start prescribing supplements, but for now we want you to understand why we refrained for so long.

Taking More Supplements And Higher Doses Does Not Equate To Better Health.

We hear all the time about the benefits of supplements for your health but if you already have enough then you don't need more. Supplements only help if you are deficient in something, so follow these three steps to understanding the benefits of supplements:

1. Get your stomach working properly to make sure you will absorb the vitamins and minerals from supplements and food. When your gut is healthy, you will need far fewer supplements.
2. Get assessed to find out if or what you are deficient in.
3. Find a customized supplement that only has what YOU need in it, in the right dose. Find a reputable company that manufactures a supplement that is specifically for you. This is a link to the trusted company we work with and use for all our Wellness Partners: **wellnessmethod.idlife.com**

Vitamins Taken In Quantities Out Of Proportion To Minerals Deplete The Body.

Interestingly enough, some of the minerals that are most easily depleted are most directly related to weight gain. Yet, there's a plethora of weight loss beverages on the market loaded with vitamins accompanied by only a minuscule amount of the critically important trace minerals we need.

6 Reasons We Are Nutrient Depleted

Here are the six primary reasons that we've deduced for mineral depletion:

1. We've moved away from eating wild foods that contain significantly higher levels of all vitamins, minerals, and essential fats.
2. Depleted soils from industrial farming and modification techniques cause animals and vegetables to have fewer nutrients.
3. Processed foods fill the grocery stores with no useable nutrients despite the "fortified with" claims.
4. The total burden of environmental toxins and chronic stress on our bodies.
5. Store bought, synthetic supplements that can't be digested and many times don't have what they claim they do on labels.
6. The supplement companies are no better than the food companies about what they have on their labels as is the case stated earlier with major companies being sued. So, finding a source you can trust is critical.

Nutrient Deficiencies, Blood Sugar And Belly Fat

Obesity and malnutrition go hand in hand. Processed, high-sugar, high-calorie foods contain almost no nutrients, yet require more vitamins and minerals to digest and metabolize them. It's a double whammy. Obesity and diabetes both stem from malnutrition. Experts describe diabetes as dehydration while in a pool of water-the sugar is everywhere, yet can't get into the cells. Your metabolism is sluggish, and the cells don't communicate. Nutrients are an essential part of correcting insulin resistance. The metabolism of fat cannot take place without the essential nutrients. Each step in every chemical reaction for fat metabolism requires the presence of specific enzymes, minerals and vitamins. Without these important substances, the ability to lose fat is impossible. Due to your unique biology, a deficiency in any of the above varies from person to person. The key is discovering **what you are lacking**. Vitamins are 'essential' for proper function, which means that they are not made inside your body and must be consumed in our diet.

Here are three ways that the right kind of supplements help metabolism:

1. They make your cells more sensitive to insulin.
2. They make you more effective at metabolizing sugar and fats.
3. Special fibers (that we will discuss in a minute) can slow the absorption of sugars and fats into the bloodstream.

This leads to a faster metabolism, more balanced blood sugar, improved cholesterol, less inflammation, fewer cravings, more weight loss, and more energy. If you have diabetes we recommend additional nutrients to reset and correct metabolic imbalances, improve insulin function, balance blood sugar, and reduce inflammation.

▶ **BIG FAT LIE: A post workout sugary, protein-filled smoothie or a sugary popular sports-aid drink is a good way to quench your thirst and recover from your workout.** Did you know that many of the sports teams that have the big sports-aid company's logo coolers on their team benches don't really have sports-aid company's logo inside of them? That's right!

▶ **Fact: The big-name sports drink company is paying for the advertising to have their names there, but most teams don't touch the stuff.** That drink is full of sugar and other harmful ingredients. You can look it up.

What Is Really Going On?

You are constantly reminded in the media of the dire state of the health of America, yet all the diet recommendations from the endless so-called experts are still not helping. Why is that? We'll tell you why: Two words: **Gut Health**

Gut Health

If you are not already, you should become familiar with these terms:

- Microbiota: the symbiotic microorganisms/bacteria of the gastrointestinal tract.
- Microbiome: the genes in your cells that make up the microbiota.

Gut atrophy and inflammation create overgrowth of organisms like candida or foreign pathogens. If you have this overgrowth, you may have been exposed to it as much as 30 years ago, but it's been dormant because the gut *was* healthy enough to cope with it. As your stress increases over the years along with gut inflammation, this causes microbial changes which allows the organism to proliferate and penetrate the stomach lining. This is called 'Leaky Gut' and this condition activates your immune system. When the immune system gets activated it often leads to autoimmune disease.

In order for nutrient balance to be restored we must start with a healthy digestive system to assimilate nutrients. There are five common causative factors of digestive dysfunction that create chronic stomach inflammation:

1. Medications: Steroids, Antibiotics, Antacids, Xenobiotics
2. Infections: H-Pylori, Yeast or Bacterial Overgrowth, Virus or Parasite
3. Stress: Increased Cortisol, increases Catecholamines
4. Hormone Imbalance: Thyroid, Progesterone, Estradiol, Testosterone
5. Neurological: Trauma, Stroke, Neuro-degeneration

The Confusion Over Vitamins, Minerals, Anti-oxidants, Fatty Acids and Amino Acids

It's frustrating to read all the conflicting studies about supplements. One day folic acid is good; the next it isn't. One day vitamin D is a lifesaver; the next day it isn't. This media whiplash is enough to make you just give up! The problem is that the studies treat nutrients like drugs. Scientists give one nutrient alone and then observe what happens. But nutrients work as a team. Broccoli is good for you and can help with many diseases, but if all you ate was broccoli, you would get sick and die because nutrients work together as cofactors to maintain balance.

Personalized Supplements And Our Approach

When we decided to bring supplements back into our practice, we wanted to ensure we were offering reputable lines that aligned with our knowledge but also took into consideration the pitfalls of the industry. In addition, the supplements had to adhere to our strict standards, so we researched and tested many companies. We investigated the makers, toured factories, and studied independent tests of their products. After a few years of this, we found a few companies we are thrilled with and meet all of our requirements! Whether you follow our recommendations or not, be sure to pick quality supplements that contain nutrients that research has shown to be beneficial to your health. Think of them as **part** of your diet, not 'in addition to' your diet. You want the best-quality food **and** the best-quality supplements going into your body!

Now that you understand what these nutrients do for your body, you might be wondering what your daily regimen should be. Everyone has unique requirements for doses, so you need to be assessed first and then find a good quality, customized supplement. After much research we invested into a platform and partner company to provide naturally sourced, whole-food, customized vitamins for our Wellness Partners. It begins with an online assessment to determine your degree of deficiencies and nutrient needs and ends with a personalized recommendation for your multivitamin regimen. Getting these ingredients in the rights dosage range for you, specifically, is important. You can go to our website to take your assessment. by going to: www.wellnessmethod.idlife.com.

We hope this provides you a better understanding about supplements and choosing the right formula for your needs. Now that you understand fat metabolism, macro and micronutrients, vitamins and minerals- you are well on your way to getting the physique you want, the health you want and the energy you've been craving! Go to it!

ACTION STEPS

What are you lacking? What are you getting too much of? Find the proper balance you need for you where you are at:

1. Macronutrients: protein, fats, carbs.
2. Micronutrients: Vitamins, Minerals, Anti-oxidants, Fiber
3. Take your personalized supplement assessment: www.mywellnessmethod.idlife.com
4. Take our Well Health Assessment on our website: www.mywellnessmethod.com
5. Customized plan: Essential nutrients for your current health status, your goals, your medications, your genetics, the seasons of the year, your height, weight, gender, stress levels, etc. .
6. Re-assessment: plan to re-assess your nutritional needs every 3 to 6 months because things change quickly.

EXERCISE

Regimen
Educational Curriculum
Coaching
Reducing Inflammation
Endocrine System
Alignment of Your Structure
Total Nutrition
Exercise

90 Minutes to Fitness After 30

I f so many Americans are exercising but are frustrated with their lack of results, what are they doing wrong? We have 57 million gym memberships in America, yet we are the most obese developed country on the planet, so how many people actually use them? A good question but the next closest country is Germany at 9 million. So, even if only half of those memberships are used we still have three times as many people working out than any other country- but still, the numbers don't lie. Obesity is an epidemic in America. When will we realize that there must be something fundamentally wrong with our current approach? Our '90 Minutes to Fitness' evolved as a response to the needs of our wellness partners for an effective workout for those with time constraints, as this is still the biggest obstacle for not exercising. There are plenty of obstacles for exercising, family, work, school, money, etc. but we've never met anyone that wasn't able to fit 90 minutes <u>a week</u> into their schedule. Yes, you read that right . . . 90 minutes per week!

There *is* a way for you to achieve lasting results from exercise, and in very little time. We listened to the feedback from hundreds of our wellness partners over the years. We learned that most programs advertised on T. V., the internet, and in magazines was either a lot of confusing hype that gave no results or just temporary results because it was just not practical in the long term for a busy schedule. We were encouraged to write this chapter to provide options that work for everyone, from those who have never worked out before all the way up to advanced exercise enthusiasts. Here are some important points we will cover along with more Big Fat Lies:

1. Aerobics is NOT the great fat burner it's advertised to be, and it will age you faster.
2. The laws of exercise physiology are universal . . . **2 Phase Training** which you will hear about later applies to everyone, male, female, young or old.
3. Muscle is the true fountain of youth and lowers your metabolic age!
4. Why sit ups are a waste of time and hurt your back.
5. Too much exercise causes catabolic stress (tearing down the body—aging your metabolism).
6. Embrace the new 'Mind Shift' that you want to lose Fat, NOT weight.
7. Muscle Failure = Muscle VICTORY! You want to GAIN muscle weight.
8. Focus on how you fit into your clothes and how you feel.

90 Minutes To Fitness After 30

From the age of about 25 for females and 28 for males, your metabolism begins to slow down. Why? Because your muscles start to atrophy (shrink) and they continue to do this for the rest of your lives. So, adding muscle steps up your metabolism with small effective steps by following the eating habits outlined in the previous chapter along with our 90 Minutes to Fitness Training Method. This 90 minutes each week is designed to challenge all the systems of your body to adapt by stimulating hormones, protein (muscle) synthesis and metabolism. This program is backed by both science and our personal experience. No more hype. Just the most effective and efficient way to step up your metabolism using the right food and the right exercises for YOU. You must change your focus on the weigh scales. It will sabotage the surefire strategy which is to burn FAT, feel stronger, more energetic and develop shapely muscles. We want to keep muscle because it <u>melts fat all day long.</u>

But before any of that happens, no one has any business starting you on an exercise program without knowing what is going on with your structural (muscles and joints) health first. There is nothing worse than starting an exercise program for 3 to 5 weeks, seeing great results, your clothes fit better, your energy is better, people are commenting on your changes and all of a sudden, your knee gives out, or your back, or your shoulder. Now all the great momentum you created comes to a crashing halt! When that happens, you get frustrated and often get depressed and then you reach for something to comfort you. Comfort foods like the sugary treats our mom gave us when we were blue or for others its alcohol, or nicotine or caffeine. Whatever the case is, we want to help you avoid this altogether, so we always start with a structural assessment from head to toe before moving anyone into exercise. We highly recommend you take this first step. Find a good body worker (chiropractor, physical therapist, massage therapist) to make certain your structure is ready for an exercise program.

Effective Exercise

Effective exercise for one person will be different for another, yet over the years we have too often seen trainers give the same generic program to everyone. Exercise must provide **catabolic stress** to your body, **catabolic** meaning tearing down muscle by inflicting microscopic tears. This catabolic stress **stimulates** the **anabolic phase** or repair and building of muscle. The anabolic process can last hours or days. Challenging exercise must stimulate the nervous system and the endocrine (hormone) system. Exercise can be destructive if done incorrectly and an excess of exercise causes too much catabolic stress (more damage than the body can repair before the next workout). The body is amazingly efficient at rebuilding and repair if the proper nutrients are available and enough rest is allowed.

Muscle = A Youthful Metabolism

Now before you work yourself into a frenzy and say, "I don't want to build muscle! I don't want to look like a body builder or the Hulk, I just want to lose weight." We are not talking about that much muscle, just a measly 3-5 pounds of muscle can make the difference for you. Adding 5 pounds of muscle is critical to fat loss; muscle that you will hardly notice. 5 pounds of muscle burns the caloric equivalent of a 2.5 mile run every day, 365 days a year! The conventional plan of riding a bike or walking for 30-60 minutes a day along with a few 'toning' exercises you found online is not working for America. Neither is the plan to put long hours in the gym which ends up unrealistic for most people to continue for the long term. You are going to learn what "metabolic burst" exercise is and why it is superior to traditional low intensity, 'cardio' exercise for health. Our love affair with low intensity cardio has got to come to an end. This type of exercise requires many hours and days every week. You can get far better results with metabolic bursts that stimulate fat burning hormones in only **90 minutes a week.**

Measuring Your Success

You should want to know how to measure your results when you are working towards changing your metabolism and adding muscle. Weight is a poor indicator of health unless it is extremely high or very low. Try not to fixate on the scale. The **Metabolic Assessment** is a critical tool to ensure you are truly burning fat, and not burning up water or muscle. This confirms that you are moving out of Fat Storing and into the Fat Burning Zone, thus ensuring that you are getting metabolically younger using 90 Minutes to Fitness.

Tracking Your Progress

There are a few measuring systems that have been around for years to track your progress for your muscle building-weight loss journey. Let's review them and then talk about a better solution.

Weight: A poor indicator of health unless it is extremely high or very low. Try not to fixate on the scale.

Body Mass Index: Overestimates body fat in anyone with a muscular build and underestimate fat in those who have lost muscle mass.

Waist To Hip Ratio: Measuring multiple sites and trying to replicate the same exact position the next time leads to inaccurate results.

Metabolic Assessment: The best solution available is a formula used to assess optimal metabolism and your **Metabolic Age**. It's easy to test and it tells us some very important markers of your health including the health of your cells, your hydration and lean muscle tissue.

MEN - 75-82%   WOMEN - 69-75%

Our Metabolic Assessment Tool can be ordered here
https://wellnessmethod.idlife. com/shop/t/categories/garmin/
smart-scale

The Real TRUTH About Calories

The calories required to build muscle are far greater than you would imagine, and it can effectively empty out fat reserves. You see protein anabolism (the building of protein from amino acids) has an enormously high energy cost. It takes approximately **45,000 calories to build a pound of muscle!** Do you see how amazing the prospect of building just 2-4 pounds of muscle can be for someone who wants to lose 20 pounds?

The First Step is to uncover what your real driving force is fueling your desire to start exercising. The fire within why you want to achieve these goals is a very powerful core element of your success. Some common reasons are:

- You've seen what obesity and disease is doing or has done, to your family or friends
- To not just 'be around' for your grandchildren, but to be able to play with and enjoy them
- You've seen the financial cost of being sick in America
- You're just sick and tired of being sick, tired and depressed
- You want more energy, more confidence and a better outlook
- You want less fat, so you can be more comfortable and fit into your clothes

Now, take a moment to answer this- What is your strategy to staying healthy for the REST OF YOUR LIFE?

Write this down and put it in a special place to keep you on track. Now, you might be saying that this is way too far ahead to think about but trust me, that is exactly why people end up in a health crisis . . . If all you're thinking about is "*I will do this for a couple months and everything will be great*", that is planning to fail. Why? Because what's the point of a yoyo approach to your health? Yes, you will see some results but for most of you the reality is you did not get to this place overnight and you aren't going to turn it around overnight. You can see big changes in 6 - 8 weeks but why not create a program that works for the long term? Where would you like to be in 6 months? How about one year? If you lost 50 pounds in 6 months would you be a happier person? No longer diabetic, would that be worthwhile? Sleeping better? Out of pain? Six months goes by in a 'blink' so, would you consider this a reasonable amount of time to see results? If so, let's work to set up short term goals first, (this is the hard part) and long-term goals (the easy part) that you can stick with.

The Startling Truth About Cardio Aerobics

In this section, you will learn about the most overrated form of weight loss: Cardio Aerobic Exercise. We have worked in the fitness industry for twenty-five years, we have owned clinics located inside of health clubs and **this BIG FAT LIE drives us crazy!**

BIG FAT LIE: Cardio/Aerobics is the best way to burn fat. If it was true we would be one of the thinnest countries in the world. Walk in to any gym during busy hours and the cardio equipment is always full! Now, yes you will lose fat doing this, but you also burn muscle! In the past 30 years gyms have exploded in America but in that same time our rates of diabetes, obesity and heart disease have doubled and tripled. You see people every day running down the street or sweating on the stair-climber and nothing changes except they begin to limp from overuse injuries or even disappear and then show up at our clinic showing us their scars from surgery.

Fact: We have helped countless wellness partners lose 40-50 pounds without cardio aerobics. In fact, we've had some lose as much as 100 pounds without cardio. Cardio is helpful for the heart and lungs, but you can get those same benefits without the injuries in a fraction of the time. Now, if you're training for marathons, that's a different story but most of us are not doing that. The truth is if you rely on cardio to lose weight you're setting yourself up for failure. So, we're not here to say "don't do any cardio"—We are saying that if you are depending on it to lose weight, you are setting yourself up for failure.

The BIG FAT Aerobics Lie Just May Kill you!

Aerobics has been promoted hard in America since 1968 when Dr. Ken Cooper published "Aerobics ". Aerobics is any continuous movement, using the larger muscles of the body, for a minimum of 20 minutes. It was considered the best fat burner and many still believe it contributes to a longer life. Take a look at the latest exercise magazines. You will find the same old, tired exercise plans. Unfortunately, the problem with this advice is, it doesn't work, and it prematurely ages you! It makes your heart and lungs more efficient, but it reduces your body's reserve capacity to handle sudden, high energy demands. This can mean the difference between surviving or dying from a heart attack. Doing aerobics for more than 10 minutes makes you more efficient which sounds good but there's a trade-off. Your cardiovascular system loses the ability to provide BURST energy, and that increases your risk of a fatal heart attack. The fact is that most heart attacks aren't from a lack of endurance, they happen when there's a **sudden, demand on your heart.** i. e. : lifting a heavy object, during sex or high emotional stress. It is theorized that the heart simply can't adapt to the sudden change in the energy demand.

We all remember the sad story of marathoner Jim Fixx, who preached that long-duration cardiovascular training was the best approach to optimal health. He practiced what he preached, right up to the moment he dropped dead of a heart attack—while running. Every year long-distance runners suffer sudden cardiac death and they have higher rates of sudden cardiac death than other athletes. Marathons have emergency stations equipped to handle heart attacks, and this risk is present regardless of culture or diet. This point is simply this: Long duration aerobics helps you go longer yet sacrifices your capacity for **sudden high energy bursts.** But, it is possible for you to have the best of both worlds by doing the **right kind** of exercise.

Here are some published studies in the most respected medical journals regarding the destruction of aerobic exercise:

- **Aerobic Exercise and Increased Heart Failure:** A breakthrough study at the Institute for Experimental Medical Research, found that low intensity/long duration aerobics involved a derangement of the **calcium/ magnesium** exchange control. This is the <u>same disease mechanism that accompanies thyroid failure, heart failure, and many chronic diseases.</u> Burst exercise did not impact the calcium/magnesium exchange.
- **The American College of Sports Medicine by Dr. Stephen Seiler:** It was found that interval exercise improved maximal cardiac outputs and facilitated quicker cardiac adjustments to changes in demand improving the heart's reserve capacity than continuous cardio/aerobic exercise.

Long Distance Cardio Athletes Are Susceptible
To Coronary Artery Disease

Scientists examined the blood of long distance runners and found that after their workout they have increased cholesterol, triglycerides, and blood clotting levels and inflammation . . . all are signs of heart **distress.** In the real world your body is designed to work in intervals; chasing kids, running upstairs, heavy lifting . . . in fact most sports are actually interval training.

You have to simulate your **hormones and your metabolism so that protein synthesis** can **build your very metabolically expensive muscle.** Muscle requires thousands of calories all day long, not just during a workout. The most effective way to health and fat loss is by building and maintaining muscle. Let us be clear: if you have hours to spend every day doing low intensity exercise you will burn calories, but the number of calories burned in a typical cardio workout is meaningless. You're going to eat those right back on at your next meal. During your workout you must impose a metabolic stimulus to your hormone system to get at your fat cells.

BIG FAT LIE: Walking is good exercise. Walking is not going to get you to your health goals, yet walking has been the go-to advice to lose weight (or recover from knee or hip surgery) for 40 years from the medical industry. Well, how is that working out for us?

Fact: Let us put walking into perspective: Unless you are severely deconditioned, walking will do nothing to stimulate a metabolic response. Now don't get me wrong, walking is a fine ACTIVITY. It is enjoyable and reduces stress, but you will not change your metabolism by walking.

A Faster Way to Burn Fat! Metabolic Burst training burns more fat in a fraction of the time. Two leading experts: Fleck, PhD and Kraemer, PhD explain how to restore energy in their book <u>Designing Resistance Training Programs</u>. In a Burst workout, the energy from ATP, (the primary energy for burst training) is exhausted in 30 seconds or less. (Larson and Davies 1970; Meyer and Terjung 1979). During recovery, there is many seconds of rapid breathing to restore oxygen back to normal which is used to aerobically replace ATP. So, during recovery you burn **fat** to restore energy.

Metabolic Bursts tap into the fat stores right from the start! The thing that distracts many experts is the focus on calories burned while exercising on 'cardio' equipment, which is prominently displayed, prodding you to keep going as if this was helping you. The fact is, unless you are doing intervals, it can take 30-45 minutes before you begin to tap into your fat reserves. You first have to deplete all blood sugar and stored sugars. This kind of workout also makes you hungry due to low blood sugar, and you will consume those calories at the next meal, negating those burned during exercise. There are some post burn effects of the exercise but it's a fraction of the burn you get from Metabolic Bursts. Now, add either the Foundation, the Correction or the In-Shape exercise plan (outlined on the following pages) to the Metabolic Bursts and the added muscle will keep your metabolism stoked 24/7.

BIG FAT LIE: Aerobics helps your cardiovascular system. This confusion is from the use of *Aerobics and Cardio to mean the same thing, when in fact they are not.* Cardio is any activity that challenges the heart and lungs. Try doing squats with a challenging weight and tell us your heart and lungs aren't pumping hard.

Fact: Studies as far back as 1975 have shown that weight training improves cardiovascular health with short rest breaks. In a 1985 study on maximal oxygen uptake (cardiovascular health) and weight training without rest, noted the same benefits as runners who trained twice as many hours. Recent studies confirm the same findings, so the fact is, YOU DON'T NEED AEROBICS! Weight training done right will improve "cardio" and lung capacity. By eliminating aerobic activity, you have more time to add muscle which is more metabolically expensive and will get your metabolism ramped up! Muscle requires thousands of calories that comes right from your fat cells. Here are more studies on the superior results of Metabolic Bursts over long slow, endurance exercise:

- **Study 1:** Divided competitive runners into two groups. Group 1: increased long-distance running. RESULTS: **loss** in speed, endurance and metabolism and **increased** Cortisol. Group 2 increased sprint training. RESULTS: **increased** speed, heart capacity and metabolism and **lowered** Cortisol.
- **Study 2:** Six sessions of sprint interval training increased muscle oxidative potential and endurance capacity in recreational athletes who did 6 sprint training sessions over 2 weeks with 1- 2 rest days. Subjects performed 4-7, full out 30 second sprints with a 4-minute rest break. Cycle endurance **increased by 100% in just 2 weeks of training!** Only 15 minutes of exercise for 2 weeks, and endurance capacity doubled! Burgomaster, et al. J Appl Physiol. Feb 2005.

A Reality Check. Do you think it is reasonable to try to include 90 minutes per week to exercise? Most are very surprised that it is even possible to see results with only 90 minutes. This chapter was written for you to debunk the big myths of exercise. It is not necessary to spend hours in the gym . . . And it is possible to see results with 90 minutes a week!

As you have learned, all exercise is not created equal. Futile exercises include working small muscles (arms and calves), walking, jogging and stability exercises like the half Bosu ball. Being overweight almost always has to do with a **slow, aging metabolism.** To stimulate your metabolism, you need muscle gains by weights that must be in the 60-70-80% of 1 repetition maximum (the most weight you can lift one time) range. Without a certain intensity, hormone changes are not stimulated for protein synthesis which requires huge amounts of calories and effectively taps into your fat cells. Now, on the other side of the coin . . . if the stimulus is too great the benefits of exercise are lowered and even negated since over training has a heavy drain on the body and negatively effects hormones to becomes counterproductive.

In our quest to really provide a user friendly, customized program that our partners could stick to, we created a giant library of Wellness Method Exercise Videos so that we can choose from a menu to help you achieve your fitness goals. We knew from our years of working in fitness, and with the months we spent refining and simplifying these videos that our wellness partners would love them, and the response has been overwhelming. The 10-15 second video clips on our member's website give you a how-to reminder of each exercise no matter what Phase of your training you are in. You can even go back to a previous phase if you are unable to exercise due to some unavoidable circumstance because life happens and sometimes we have to step back. But that is no reason to stop. We are like a personal trainer that is always on the clock for our Wellness Partners: whenever they need a quick review or a complete re-start, we are just a click away on our website or in their email inbox.

You now know all exercise is not created equal and you also learned that you can actually over train the body which will negatively affect your hormone levels and become counter-productive to your health goals. Keeping this in mind, this is where 2 Phase Training really shines.

2 Phase Training can be accomplished in as little as 90 minutes a week. It is so effective because it combines all the essential exercises that you need for a healthy, youthful metabolism into 2 simple phases:

2 Phase Training: Reset Your Metabolic Age to Reclaim Your Youth

PHASE 1: *Metabolic Bursts*

The best technique to burn body fat. Interval training taps into fat burning immediately and as studies have proven will burn 9 times the fat that aerobics can burn in the same time frame. Intervals have a positive effect on heart reserve as opposed to conventional long duration, low intensity cardiovascular exercise.

This phase of training burns fat for up to **three hours** after a 20-30-minute session. Compared to cardio/aerobics which has a post-fat burn of just a few minutes. Keep in mind that we created this program for those with time constraints, knowing that performing 90 minutes per week will produce results. . . . but if you want to get faster results you have a couple of options: Add a 3rd In-SHAPE workout in (explained below), providing it is a different body part from the previous In-SHAPE workout.

Important Note: High intensity is a relative term. Output that might be high intensity for one person might seem an easy cruise for another. As you become better conditioned, increase the intensity if you're pacing yourself a little. IT'S THAT SIMPLE. This is by far more effective than low intensity AEROBICS at burning fat and much more fun!

Pro Tip: Would you like to increase your results by 300% **Do your Metabolic Bursts when you first get up in the morning before eating.**

The Fat-Burning Zone

This Big Fat Lie has inundated the fitness industry for decades and it needs to cease! The theory of the Target Heart Rate or Fat Burning Zone suggests that once your heart rate is out of the "fat-burning zone," you cease to burn fat and start to burn carbohydrates instead. Low intensity exercise will first burn sugar stored in muscles as the first source of energy. Once sugar is used up the body starts burning fat. The time it takes to tap into the fat cells is different for everyone, but 45 minutes is the average so don't eat carbs before exercise, and if possible do aerobic exercise first thing in the morning before eating. Carbs MUST first be used before you switch to fat for energy.

Here is why Metabolic Bursts works

1. After an overnight 8-12 hour fast, your body's stores of glycogen are depleted, and you burn more fat when glycogen is low.
2. Eating causes a release of insulin. Insulin interferes with the mobilization of body fat.
3. There is less carbohydrate (sugar) in your blood after an overnight fast. With less sugar available you burn more fat.
4. If you eat immediately before a workout, you have to burn what you just ate before tapping into stored body fat (and insulin is elevated after a meal).

PHASE 2: *Resistance Training*

We divided this section into three categories based on your fitness level and ability.

2a. The Foundation The foundation is designed to wake your muscles up from their slumber.

2b. The Correction A program to correct muscle imbalances leading to injury.

2c In-SHAPE (**St**imulating **H**ormones **a**nd **P**rotein **E**xpression) The emphasis is on using the larger muscles to stimulate hormones and protein synthesis which is very metabolically expensive and taps into **fat stores** during the recovery process.

Phase 2a: The Foundation

A thorough full-body program in a short rest fashion, designed to be an introduction to weight training to wake up deconditioned muscles. It minimizes micro-trauma to muscles and joints and reduces post exercise soreness all combined to have a positive effect on staying with the program.

The First Step

Before you start the Foundation, be certain that you have inflammation under control as we covered in the Alignment section of this book. If inflammation cannot be controlled through home care, consult a specialist. The Foundation is a thorough full body introduction to weights. Our experience for over 25 years has shown us that the beginner, the de-conditioned and the senior, all benefit from a full-body wake up call. It prepares you not only physically, but psychologically, for the challenges in the next phase that will pull your body into proper alignment. Without the Foundation injuries are far more likely to occur.

Beginning Your Foundation

Start the Foundation of your workout with a very comfortable resistance. i. e. if you're going to do squats then do a squat with a light weight for a warm-up. We are going to be performing total body workouts, using all the largest muscles of the body at each workout. Therefore, we are going to perform at least one warm-up set for all the major muscle groups and include a few core exercises to stabilize the area for the workout. The Foundation exercises should be completed at a steady pace, moving from one exercise to the next without rest other than the time it takes to make adjustments to the machines or weights you are using. The movements are performed **slowly so as to feel** the muscles being worked, linking the mind - body connection. We use the foundation to teach beginners the awareness of their muscles and joints and how to engage them. Always initiate exercise with muscles, no jerking movement or momentum. We are going to give you an overview as we cannot prescribe your program for you specifically without meeting you or speaking with you.

How to Select the Best Weight

When starting out lifting weight, we know you might be thinking, "Where do I start?" Everyone reading this book will be at a different fitness level, so there will be some trial and error. Always err on the side of lighter weight to avoid injury. It won't take you long to determine a challenging weight to perform 10-15 repetitions. For each exercise, select a weight that you can barely get 10-15 repetitions (reps) done. If you can do more than 15 reps, then increase weight, if you can't do at least 10, then lower the weight. Don't get caught up in worrying about how much weight you're using. The goal is the right resistance to match the right number of reps. Those that get caught up increasing weight too soon lose focus on good form which leads to a weak foundation, injuries and plateaus.

Supersets

A superset is two exercises completed back to back with no rest between other than the time it takes to adjust the weight. The two exercises will usually be antagonistic to each other, that is, if you are performing a pushing exercise first in the superset, the second exercise will be a pulling movement.

Reps (Repetitions)

A Rep is the number of times you do the particular movement. Do your reps at approximately a 2-second concentric (lifting) movement and at a 3 or 4 second eccentric (lowering) movement. Slowing down the eccentric part of the movement slows your momentum and targets the muscle. It's important to always keep control of the movement to avoid risk of injury.

Phase 2b: The Correction

You will be ready to move on to the corrective exercise phase of your program once finished with The Foundation. A split routine that uses compound exercises in a giant set fashion. Beginners find these compound movements to be inherently more comfortable to perform as you align your body for good posture, coordination and balance. As always, we recommend checking in with a good structural doctor/therapist to assess muscle imbalances. As you move into the correction phase you might be wondering "What is Structural Balance?" This question was thoroughly answered in the Alignment Chapter of this book. The specific exercises needed are going to be different for everyone depending on their specific structural imbalances, so you will need to see a type of structural doctor or therapist to address this concern. The most common people to work with on this are chiropractors, osteopaths, physical therapists, massage therapists and personal trainers that have advanced certifications. We have a list of references on our website depending on your area.

Phase 2c: To Be In SHAPE requires Stimulating Hormones and Protein Exercises

This challenging split routine uses a wide variation of movements in a giant set fashion based on your ability and your fitness goals. In addition to giving your body shape and contour, muscle increases your metabolism and burns fat around-the-clock. Now before you jump to conclusions, we are not referring to the excessive bodybuilder look. What we are talking about is shape and curves that most people are happy to have. Now the good part - gaining that kind of muscle is rather simple and the truth is, most people work much too hard and long trying to develop shapely muscles. What we've been telling you should feel like a breath of fresh air. You see, developing tone and shape has been hyped-up by endless fitness selling gimmicks on late night infomercials or memberships salesmen at fitness clubs, as THE SOLUTION to a toned and shapely body. You've been misled and we are hear to clear things up for you!

Giant Sets

These are not new to experienced trainers in the world of sports medicine, however, you won't find them in fitness magazines or on TV. Remember, exercise is 'big business' and they do not want to lose you as a customer! 90 Minutes to Fitness is well documented in medical journals but more importantly, it WORKS! A Giant Set is four exercises completed back to back with no rest between other than the time it takes to adjust the weight. For our purposes, these four exercises will typically be arranged so that you work one muscle as you work another that is in opposition. So, if you are performing a pushing exercise first in the set, the second exercise will be a pulling movement. Although you should have a good idea after training a few times as to what weight to use on the first giant set, your strength will vary slightly from workout to another. The giant set allows you to adjust the resistance allowing you to reach muscle failure which = Success! Giant Sets turn up the intensity by performing four opposing muscle groups back to back and challenging the body, to step up your cardio—pulmonary response and burn more calories! This creates a time efficient workout. The effectiveness of the Giant Sets is based on the following;

- Use larger muscles of the body
- Perform exercise with no rest breaks
- Exercise 2-3 days a week
- Perform the last set to failure

One of the Biggest, Fattest Lies sold to the average person, is that it takes hours and hours to build shapely, strong muscles and this is simply not true if you are using the larger muscles (chest, back and legs) as opposed to the smaller muscles (biceps, triceps and calves). We call the exercises using the small muscles, 'wimpy exercises' since they don't stimulate **metabolism or hormones**. So, replace wimpy exercises like leg extensions with multi-joint movements like squats. Replace the basic lateral raises with shoulder press, bicep curls with seated rows, etc. Heavier resistance stimulates metabolism and hormones. Our goal is to step up your metabolism, not build biceps! Putting the large muscles to work is the best way to do that. All these techniques combine to create a challenge to the body down to the cellular level. Remember, the recovery and repair process caused by these workouts, requires a massive calorie expense that comes from . . . your fat cells! Because this is so efficient, you only need a limited number of sets.

Free Weights vs. Weight Machines

There are many options to consider when it comes to exercise equipment and there are pros and cons to each. Free weights and cables are simpler and allow for considerable movement freedom. Machines force you to move along a predetermined path dictated by the machine design. Machines limit the stabilizer and synergistic muscles of the body, but machines still challenge large muscles and stimulate metabolism, hormones, and protein synthesis. Muscles don't know whether you're doing a push-up, a machine bench press, or a free weight bench press, all stressing the same muscles. Machines have a place in exercise especially for beginners, the deconditioned and balance challenged.

Training The CORE

Core muscles includes the abdominals, the obliques, the lower back and upper thigh muscles. Working the core muscles will rev up your metabolism. The main functions of the core are to provide strength to protect your spine and pelvis which provide the base for all body movement. To focus only on crunches will create imbalances in your core. When you twist using the obliques (side muscles), you also train the rectus abdominis (6-pack muscle).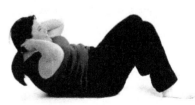

Why Sit-Ups Don't Work

We have watched sit ups performed inefficiently for years because abdominal muscles work in only 30% of the movement through a sit-up. 70% of the muscle work done in a sit-up does not come from the abdominals. Sit ups past 30 degrees engage the hip flex or (iliopsoas) muscles and injure the spine. They run from the front of your upper leg, through the pelvis, up to the lower six vertebrae. When they contract, they pull your upper body to your legs—just as your abs do but the psoas has a huge range of motion. Activating the psoas muscle causes your vertebrae to grind together. The psoas works when your legs are extended, or your feet are being held. When doing Sit-Ups, the psoas competes with your abs in the first 1/3 of the movement. The abs take over in the last 2/3's of movement. With each contraction, the psoas tugs on your spine causing you to arch and compress your vertebrae to grind together leading to pain and disk degeneration.

This is why we advocate the 'crunch' which is safer and more effective. But the problem with the crunches is they are not metabolically effective, yet people do hundreds of them hoping for a smaller midsection. This time could be far better spent.

Attention Ladies: How to Tone Your Buttocks, Thighs, Lower Abs

What holds many females back from reaching their potential is the fear of building muscles. Ladies - weight training cannot, will not and can never make you big and bulky unless your goal is body building. Exercise causes muscle to stay toned and gives you a pleasing, curvy shape. Our response to women who are afraid of gaining muscles is this: Many of you believe you are getting bigger at the onset of a weight training program. When you begin exercising, the butt muscles, thighs and back of the arms are often flaccid, or saggy because, no exercise means soft flabby muscles. . . . . Are you with us so far? After just 2 to 4 weeks of training your muscles will perk up and you will start to lose body fat and reduce your size. Remember- the goal of any effective fat loss program is to increase your metabolism, so you must add muscle! Muscle is very dense, so you will hardly notice a couple pounds of calorie burning muscle. Let us ask you an important question- Would you trade 20 pounds of fat for 2 or 3 pounds of muscle? You better be saying yes!

What You Need to Know About Stretching

Recent studies on stretching show that pre-exercise stretching has little effect on preventing injuries and may inhibit performance. Don't stretch cold muscles, it makes no sense. The warm up goal is to increase muscle temperature. As muscles warm-up your blood flows and joints get lubricated. A growing body of research shows that stretching before sports like football, soccer, running, etc., is actually counterproductive. One study showed a 28% drop in muscle contraction. Strength requires tension and stretching can deactivate tension as well as create the potential to harm joints by over stretching. The emphasis for the de-conditioned beginner should be on strength and protecting joints since the deconditioned already have loose joints from their sedentary lifestyle. Prioritize what you really need from an exercise program and focus your time there. If you are flexible enough to perform your normal daily routine without pain or restriction, you don't need extra stretching. Muscle pain or other joint problems should be assessed by a professional and prescribed stretches may be applied. Athletes often require sport specific stretches to improve performance however, all stretching should follow after training when the body is warm, so it does not affect muscle force during competition.

Plateaus

Overtraining is the biggest mistake made by beginners and advanced athletes. The body is only capable of handling so much catabolic stress (tearing down of muscle) and then it must be allowed recovery time. If you don't recover between workouts your body fatigues and fat increases from the loss of muscle. This condition of being **fatigued**

and not making any improvements in your workout is often labeled as **a plateau** when in reality it may be overtraining. How do most people respond to plateaus? By doing more of course! They step up their training, making it even harder for the body to repair from all the overtraining. Do you get the picture yet? More training is not the answer. **Intense training with the right amount of recovery is essential.**

Overtraining And Adrenal Exhaustion

It should be apparent that there is a lot of wasted of time and effort on exercise. There is no denying the motivation and discipline of millions of Americans, but unfortunately, they never achieve their goals following the big fat lies of exercise. This often leads to overtraining, fatigue and fat retention. You can test yourself to see if you are doing too much volume before you start your training. Check your resting pulse first thing in the morning before you get out of bed and log how many beats in 60 seconds. Do this for three consecutive days to establish **your base line.** After you train for a few weeks, check your morning pulse again. If you pulse is **5 to 10 points higher** than your initial base line, this is a strong indicator of overtraining. Take a few days off and do not return to doing the exercise until your morning pulse returns to the base line for two days. For example, let's say you find your initial morning pulse over three days is 68. This is considered your baseline. Let's say you do a random check and find your pulse is 73. This indicates you should not train that day and should wait until your baseline pulse is back to 68.

Health Club Or Home Workouts

We are often asked if it is possible to get a good workout at home and we always answer yes. You will not have the variety a health club offers however, but if it means the difference between exercise and no exercise because of time or other reasons, by all means a home workout has many benefits and in fact, our website has a wealth of information on home workouts.

ACTION STEPS

An exercise program only works if you do it consistently. You could have the best equipment, best trainer, but it must be **realistic for your lifestyle** if you are going to stick with it. So why do people who are motivated begin a program and then quit? They did not set themselves up to succeed. The solution is to create a plan that you can stick with by following these steps:

1. Customized Plan: Assess what level you are at. The Foundation, The Correction or the SHAPE workout.
2. Make a plan to ensure you are doing the essential exercises for your health status, your goals, gender, lifestyle, etc. You may like to play tennis, swim, hike, and that is fine. We don't want to take that away but, you now understand the science of how to reset a slow metabolism that will change your health.
3. Re-assessment: Plan to re-assess your fitness every 3 to 6 months because your body adapts to exercise after awhile so to ensure you are getting **Results!** If you are investing time and energy without getting your desired results, you will get frustrated or bored and quit. But if you get good results it keeps you going and a new plan keeps things fresh.
4. Avoid These Common Mistakes:

   - Poor Timing: Even when highly motivated, priorities such as children, work, school, etc. do not leave much time for long hours of exercise.

- Same generic program: Many trainers want to fit clients into their program rather than creating a program to fit the individual.
- Confusing and Too Complex: Frustrating and hard to follow is what we hear a lot.
- Overtraining: The overachievers quit from exhaustion and again, no results. Motivation gets you started. Results keep you going!

5. Where To Exercise? At a gym? Your home? A park? The best results happen when you leave home and remove yourself from distractions. Google the gyms in the area and find something convenient and cost friendly.

6. Occupy Your Brain: Find something interesting to listen to! We have a plethora of things to choose from. We like to listen to inspiring speakers to workout our mind as our body gets fit. Music, audiobooks . . . you have the whole internet at your fingertips.

7. Mind Shift Your "Mind Set": The epiphany that it does not require long hours of exercise to see results will allow you to make exercise a part of your life. This gimmick free approach helps you stay in a positive mind set without the long hours required by other programs. You can achieve your goals with 90 minutes per week and the results drive the mind which drives the body. You won't feel the stress to exercise 6 days a week, which can cause the body to hold on to fat. The new psychology helps reinforce that with just **90 minutes to Fitness** on a regular basis, you can achieve your goals.

HAVE FUN with it and enjoy the process!

CHAPTER 10

A NEW ERA OF HEALTHCARE HAS FINALLY ARRIVED

"It is more important to treat the person who has the disease, than the disease that the person has."

~ *William Osler, father of 20th century medicine*

Congratulations! You now know more about health and vitality than 90% of the general population. If you're still reading this book, it is clear you're serious about your health. You've learned that the existing, medical model is driven by symptom management and profit. On April 16, 2018 it was widely reported that Goldman Sachs was asked in a biotech research report: "Is Curing Patients A Sustainable Business Model?" Companies are in business to make a profit and we have no problem with that, but not when it comes to health. ***When lives are on the line, the bottom line should not be the over-riding factor.*** In America, we make up 5% of the world's population but we use 75% of pharmaceuticals. We have more diseases prevalent today than at any other time in our history.

Functional Medicine should be accessible to everyone and it needs to be reported on CNN, 20/20, Oprah, all the majors. It needs to be front page news and on the covers of Newsweek and Time. Our government should fund research and courses in Functional Medicine and it should be available for all levels in healthcare. Millions are suffering needlessly and dying because our system maintains the status quo and perpetuates the insurance care model. We are committed to increasing the momentum around this approach and creating a tipping point so that everyone can utilize this approach. We have been referred to as 'Shining Lights' by our Wellness Partners and colleagues. We don't say that to brag, we say it to create momentum. Through the results that we get with our Wellness Partners, and through this book, we are telling the world about the incredible potential of The Wellness Method, but we can't do it alone. We need to increase our ever-growing community and we'd like to invite you to be a part of it. First, we want to encourage you to adopt our methods and in addition we recommend you find a functional medicine practitioner that can support you. Then, it is our greatest hope that you will be a walking example, like so many before you, of what is possible when we learn how to focus on our health. By working together, we have the power to create a tremendous change in the lives of so many and in our broken healthcare system. *If each of you share the information you learned in this book, we can start a grassroots community for change.*

A Note From Dr. Kobsar

"Where can I find a doctor who practices the way that you do?" That was the question I was recently asked when giving a talk about our Wellness Method to a group of public health educators who deal with all the leading-edge nutritional and medical advice. They are the key decision and policy makers in our government offices. They are the top thinkers, creative leaders and very connected to the health world.

Yet they were asking me for help to find a doctor! Unfortunately, this is a question that I hear over and over when I speak about healthcare that deals with the roots of illness, not just the symptoms. Everybody wants it, but nobody can find it. I am working on many exciting initiatives, such as the creation of a fellowship training program, and collaborating on groundbreaking research on Wellness and Functional Medicine, so we're making progress. But it can be challenging to find qualified practitioners who truly understand this model and it astounds me that even though 125 million Americans suffer with chronic disease, they still can't find someone with proper training that can truly help them.

I was lucky enough to be in the early development of Functional Wellness Medicine during my years at my County's Hospital System, where I had the benefit of a truly amazing leadership group who were willing to explore this new medicine with me. It was through their visionary leadership that I was first introduced to working with severe chronic disease conditions and learn from the metabolic tests that allowed me to see deep into the roots of their illness. It was through these experiences that I gained the knowledge to help so many people for which symptom-based medicine fails. Here is one final story of one of them.

Case Study: 5 CD4-cells

I remember a patient that was referred to me who struggled for years with HIV, chronic fatigue, irritable bowel syndrome, depression, arthritis, sinusitis, severe muscle pain and brain fog. He also had a 50-pound loss of muscle mass which led to prescription anabolic steroids and growth hormones with the added side effect of causing diabetes. He also was down to only five CD4-cells in his entire body. CD4 cells are the primary cells that you use to fight infections and when people have a chronic disease the CD 4 cells are working to save our lives. The normal amount of these is 400- 1600 in one cubic millimeter of blood. He had five IN HIS ENTIRE BODY. So, he did what only he would and named them! What can you say about a person that is in this kind of a place and still is able to still have the strength to make light of the situation and name his last 5 remaining CD4 cells?! He was taking medication to treat symptoms and when he entered our Wellness Program we worked together over many months to show him how to address the causes of his symptoms. We dealt with his gut dysfunction, detoxified him, fixed his mitochondria to restore cell metabolism and energy production and addressed the inflammation raging through his body. Just one year later, he was a new person and his CD4 counts were at 1000 and climbing. He reduced his medications and even came to work for us as a volunteer fitness trainer because he would not let me pay him. He wanted to help others in similar situations get better. And that started a huge influx of patients that came to volunteer because they wanted to jump in and help. Soon I had a whole team of former patients that became trainers. Eventually he was released from disability and went back to work, 50 pounds heavier in health, without diabetes, depression, pain, fatigue, and digestive problems. He had his life back after 10 years of suffering.

As we face the tsunami of chronic diseases that will cost our global economy $47 trillion over the next twenty years. As we spend more and more for health care, we get less and less. Chronic diseases affect one in two Americans and accounts for 80 percent of our health care costs. We need a different model to beat this epidemic. If you begin with the education in this book and implement the actions steps provided, here is what's possible for you: Close your eyes and picture yourself 4 weeks from today. What day will that be? Got it in your mind? Great . . . Just 28 days from now, you look in your bathroom mirror. It's the same mirror, but it has a brand-new reflection. The 'you' that's looking back has less inflammation, a younger metabolic age and a smile of pride and hope for the future. Compliments from your friends and loved ones who are happy for what you've accomplished . . . and most important, <u>you're happy with yourself.</u> You've re-programmed your metabolism and added a new shape and muscle tone and you rest easier at night.

Is Wellness Method For Everyone?

Not if you are okay with taking medications for the rest of your life and the unwanted side effects that go with them. Let us be very clear, we are not trying to convince anyone of anything. The Wellness Method is only for those that are looking for something different then what is already available in the health care system. The Wellness Method is a unique blueprint for health based on the RECREATE principals that you now hold in your hand. All you have to do now is take action. We know you will!

ACTION STEPS:

1. You have the rest of your life in this body, so how do you want to live? Where do you start? Well, you finished the book, hopefully you took the action steps. If you haven't taken all the steps, why not? If not now, when?

2. Find credible resources for your wellness education. They can be books, webinars, courses, etc. . . . . If you are unsure where to find credible resources, feel free to contact us!

If you have taken steps, then we want you to be part of this community of people that made the same important decision to focus on their health. If our approach makes sense to you, we'd like to support you in your health journey. Here are a few ways you can participate:

How to contact Wellness Method

Here are a few different ways you can connect with us:

1. Join our Facebook community at https://www.facebook.com/drkobsar/
2. Take a free health assessment at wellnessmethod.idlife.com
3. Watch one of our webinars. Email your request to info@mywellnessmethod.com
4. View our website and the many testimonies from our Wellness Partners: mywellnessmethod.com

THE END

or . . .

YOUR BEGINNING

"I'm trying to free your mind, Neo.
But I can only show you the door.
You're the one that has to walk through it".

Morpheus, The Matrix Film, 1999

WARNING: SCIENCE NERD ALERT!

W e spent a lot of time deliberating, discussing, hashing out, going back and forth and . . . well, let's just say we had some heated debates as to whether or not we should include this chapter. We both felt it was important information, but one of us felt it was a little too much clinical information and would be out of place in the context of this book. And one of us felt that though clinical, it was too important to leave out. We'll let you guess who was on which side of this discussion :). But in the end we both felt it was important to include, so enjoy!

For those that are curious, this is **a deep dive into body systems and functional medicine** that definitely crossed over into territory reserved for science enthusiasts. But we live in Silicon Valley and there are a lot of Dr. Kobsar type of people that come with a strong science background. As you can see, we compromised and found a good place for it as an optional read for those that want to buckle up, put on the thick plastic glasses, pocket protectors and bring your hunger to learn more about how your body systems work!

A SYSTEMS APPROACH TO OPTIMAL HEALTH:

Have you ever seen a bored newborn? Of course not. Babies radiate awe, joy, wonder, vitality, energy, life, and rejuvenation. It's their natural state. But it's your natural state too. You are always in touch with the magic of life. Even the most ill person retains a healing ability: cut their skin, they'll bleed 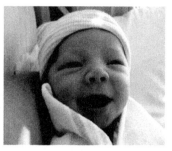 *and begin healing. If there's life, there's still a spark of healing, of hope. This incredible ability you have to heal, and auto-regulate body functions is due to an inner intelligence that you are born with. Dr. Lewis Thomas, M. D. said," A kind of super intelligence exists in each of us, infinitely smarter and possessed of technical know-how far beyond our present understanding. This is the inborn wisdom of your body. "*

—Excerpt from Dr. Kobsar's article in
Pathways to Health, August 2017

This intelligence allows your body to constantly adapt to its ever-changing environments. It knows how to digest your food without you thinking about it. It heals a cut on your finger (no, your Band-Aid doesn't do the healing), it keeps your heart beating, and it kicks up your immune system when your body is invaded by bacteria. Inborn intelligence resides everywhere in your body. It is mediated by your brain, which communicates with every muscle, gland, organ and cell in your body via your nervous and hormone system. Because your brain and the rest of your nervous system mediate your innate intelligence, it stands to reason that this system must be optimized to its highest potential if true health is to be achieved. Your nervous system really is your master computer. It regulates all functions of the body every second of your life. When it's out of sync, you're out of sync.

Emerging evidence is proving that most chronic illness is caused by the biological *reaction* to an injury, and not the initial injury. For example, melanoma can be caused by sun exposure that occurred decades earlier, and post-traumatic stress disorder (PTSD) can occur years after a bullet wound has healed. If healing is incomplete between injuries, more severe disease will result. If a new head injury is sustained before complete healing of an earlier concussion, the clinical severity of the second injury is amplified, and recovery is prolonged. This occurs even when the energy of the second impact was less than the first. Progressive dysfunction with recurrent injury after incomplete healing occurs in all organs, not just the brain. So, chronic disease results when cells are caught in a repeating cycle or loop of incomplete recovery and re-injury, unable to fully heal.

Many syndromes including Fibromyalgia, Chronic Fatigue, Multiple Sclerosis and Post Traumatic Stress are described in medical journals. A shortcoming in the explanations for all syndromes is that they fail to measure the total Allostatic Overload as the mediator between stress and disease. They also limit the application of all the body's systems. By nature, systems are complex, multi-causal, dynamic and interdependent. All of this poses an impossible challenge to insurance based, symptom care which our current healthcare model provides. Systems Medicine looks at the body where all the networks of our biology, physiology and biochemistry interact like a symphony of musical instruments playing in a harmony of health. When out of balance, this process creates disease. Systems Medicine takes all the puzzle pieces of science, all the research about how we get well and what makes us get sick and organizes it into a logical story, a story that has the capability to solve our health care crisis AND health crisis nearly overnight if it was initiated broadly. Medicine is the youngest science and there is no theory of medicine or principles that helps us navigate through chronic disease. Systems or Functional Medicine is the biggest breakthrough in medicine since the discovery of germs and antibiotics. It is a cataclysmic shift in our view of biology.

Cell Communication

Chronic illness results when cell signals malfunction, which puts a block on your healing systems. When injury happens, we see the following two events: Healing and the **Cell Danger Response (CDR)**. The CDR is a change in the use of fuel, repair, defense, signaling and recovery. The CDR is coordinated by the cell nucleus, mitochondria which are signaled by cell receptors and signal molecules. ie; serotonin, melatonin, acetylcholine, glutamate, aspartate, glycine, GABA, dopamine, norepinephrine, epinephrine, histamine, anandamide, and adenosine. All chronic diseases produce systems abnormalities that either block communication or send alarm signals between cells and tissues. Cells that can't communicate normally with other cells, are stranded from the whole and cannot integrate into normal function. They are lost, even when they are surrounded by cells. If the block in cell-to-cell communication continues, two outcomes occur:

1. Children; affects development and leads to altered function of the organs, microbiome, metabolism and immune system.
2. Adults; organ function deteriorates, more and more cells are disabled, signal malfunctions grow and health degenerates.

When stress exceeds repair, abnormal cell communication activates both the Healing Cycle and Damage Cycles.

The Healing Cycle combines wakeful activity with restorative sleep. This cycle includes balanced, integrated, and periodic use of all three energy systems of the mitochondria; glycolysis, aerobic glycolysis, and oxidative phosphorylation. Health requires brain coordination of organ function and whole body metabolism using nerve and hormone systems. Wakeful activity, locally grown, season-appropriate diet, consumed during daytime hours has been disrupted by unseasonal food availability, by the increase in night shift work and by the decline of outdoor activity- all of which has put new pressure on our genes. Modern technology helps us better understand the importance of diets that occurs naturally with the seasons and occasional short fasts to promote health throughout the year (Mattson et al. Nat. Rev. Neurosci., 2018).

The Damage Cycle OR Cell Danger Response (CDR)

Stage 1/CDR1 is devoted to damage control, innate immunity, intruder and toxin detection, inflammation and clean up.

- Triggers: bacteria, viruses, fungi, protozoa, toxins, cell disorganization (entropy), disrupted gap junctions that connect cell functions

Stage 2/CDR2 supports cell growth for replacement and tissue formation for specific organ tissue function. Each tissue has an optimum number of different cells that are needed for healthy function.

- Triggers: When cells die, they must be replaced or organs will malfunction. Stem cells are recruited to replace dead cells and to help close wounds or 'wall-off' infection with scar tissue.

Stage 3/CDR3. begins when cells begin to differentiate to take on organ-specific functions along with rebuilding, adaptive immunity, detoxification, metabolic memory, sensory and pain modulation, and sleep habits. Adjustments in gene expression, cell structure and metabolism to adapt to existing tissue conditions.

Your Body is a Self-Healing, Self-Regulating Organism

Without healing, life does not exist. Without healing, one injury predisposes to another, leading to chronic disease, accelerated aging and death. Your body was designed to heal itself. As shared in earlier chapters, every 90 days you get a brand-new liver! Your liver cells die off in that 3 months and are replaced by new ones. Every four months all your blood cells are also replaced. And before the end of the year, nearly all of you is replaced physically! This process continues, year after year, for your entire life. Although the nature of healing seems obvious from daily cuts, scrapes, and the common cold, the extension of this as a theory to explain chronic disease has only recently become possible.

The point is that your body is in a constant mode of renew and repair. However, to do this it must follow an exact program that was set in motion nearly from the time you were conceived. So, if you're not well, it stands to reason that your body is unable to follow the program. The Systems approach creates incredible hurdles for experimental research to observe changes in a laboratory setting, so unfortunately, scientists and doctors will only use a "Systems" explanation as a last resort after the symptom care model has failed.

Reframing the process of chronic illness as a systems problem that *maintains* disease, rather than focusing on remote trigger(s) that *caused* the initial injury, allows new research to focus on therapies to *unblock* the healing cycle, and restore health.

Understanding Allostatic Overload is critical to helping and allowing the body to heal. The one underlying theme of all the different syndromes (Fibromyalgia, Chronic Fatigue, etc.) is your body is left with a negative sum total of energy. Let us explain:

The systems of your body work like a simple math equation: 'Energy expended plus energy produced'. (Do NOT mistake energy for calories! As we have learned some types of calories steal your energy!) If you are optimally well, your body will expend less energy to operate its systems than what you produce from your systems. At the end of the day you will have a positive amount of energy produced and your systems are thriving. Reduced mitochondrial oxidative phosphorylation and altered structure are fundamental features of aging. The changes in aging are similar to changes that occur during the stages of the cell danger response for healing (Naviaux, 2014).

Allostasis literally means "stability through change". When you are in Allostatic Stress Overload, your body is expending more energy than it is producing. You are using more energy than you are creating and you are left with a negative amount of energy produced. This results in chronic wasting, atrophy and degeneration. Simply put, your body is wasting, shrinking and deteriorating. We can't change our genes, but we can certainly prevent Allostatic Stress Overload which leads to heart disease, cancer, diabetes, and more. When we control Allostatic Overload, we have a great opportunity to disrupt ANY chronic disease. The following four system processes are critical in the body's path to either health or disease and are a crucial part of this systems view to healing:

1. **Homeostasis:** taught in medical schools, that in order to preserve life you must stabilize your physiology with the idea of a specific 'optimum set point' for body temperature, energy balance, blood sugar, cholesterol, etc.
2. **Allostasis:** uses biological evolution and adaptation to environment, to maintain optimal health by modulating changes of the Hypothalamic-Pituitary- axis hormones, the ANS, CNS neurotransmitters inflammatory system and immune systems.

3. **Allostatic Overload (STRESS):** The consequences of draining our resources on adapting to long term stress causes disease from an energy crisis and mitochondrial dysfunction. This is the classic stress response of alarm, resistance and recovery.

4. **Hormesis:** When stress is beneficial, even lifesaving in the case of saber tooth tiger threats. It is small enough and it is turned off before an energy crisis.

The Homeostasis Model Failed. Over 50% of adults and 30% of children and teens in the United States now live with a chronic illness. Allostasis allows all organ systems to vary within a large dynamic range according to environmental changes. The range of change is very large in the young but shrink with age. ie; blood pressure in a man measured 110/70 for many hours but dropped to 90/55 during a nap. It then increased to 140/80 while preparing to go to work and dropped to 70/40 while asleep and to 50/30 for 1 h during deep sleep. (Sterling and Ever, Handbook of Life Stress, Cognition, and Health, 1988, 629-649).

Allostasis states that each blood pressure is "normal" for the changing conditions, however, if high blood pressure remains over time, then blood vessels thicken and increased blood pressure is needed to maintain blood flow. Sterling and Eyer point out that unpredictable environmental stress creates addiction in the brain to systems and signaling molecules (hormones, neurotransmitters, cytokines, and metabokines) needed for arousal and the anticipation (worry) stress response become normal. This complicates treatment and often results in 'withdrawal' symptoms, making a return to health impossible without a change in lifestyle.

With Allostatic Overload (AO), homeostasis falls in the face of stress, and disease results. Analysis of 23 measures of 7 body systems that regulate stress found that AO is a valid explanation for the adjustments from stress (Wiley et al. Psychosom. Med. 2016, 290-

301). Interestingly, all the metabolic, inflammatory, neuroendocrine, and gene expression changes that respond to stress are regulated by mitochondria (Picard et al Proc. Natl. Acad. Sci. 2015). McEwen postulates that if the mitochondria coordinates the stress response in cells activated by AO, it is the link to regulating AO and chronic disease. (Picard et al. Psychosom. Med., 2017).

System Communication

The identification of the **metabolic syndrome** was a good first step by scientists to assess chronic disease from a multi-factorial, dynamic, multi-system view rather than the conventional one system approach. i. e. : cardiovascular system, hormone system, nervous system. The first definition of metabolic syndrome was presented in 1998 as a constellation of interconnected biological, chemical and metabolic factors that increase the risk of heart disease, diabetes and death. The problem with looking at health markers like inflammation, blood pressure and heart rate, is that they only look at one point in time. This is a very limited way of looking at complex systems. The allostatic stress associated with Metabolic Syndrome is a state of ongoing inflammation caused by cumulative changes in your metabolism, your genes and your environment. Attempts have been made to expand the metabolic syndrome because the current view falls short of addressing hormones system, digestion, your immune and nervous system.

As we treat the rising tsunami of chronic disease with using acute care medicine, a growing body of literature is showing that chronic disease is a whole body disease—a *systems problem*—that won't be solved using the old paradigm. For example:

1. Autism, bipolar disorder, schizophrenia, Parkinson, and Alzheimer disease each affect the brain, but have system malfunctions that can be measured in the blood and urine.

(Gevi et al., 2016; Autism). (Han et al, 2017; Movment Disorder) (He et al., 2012, Translational Psychiatry), (Varma et al., 2018), (Yoshimi et al., 2016 BBA Clinical).

2. Rheumatoid arthritis affects joints, but also has abnormalities in the blood that show an activated Cell Danger Response (Naviaux, 2014, Translational Psychiatry) for years before the onset of joint disease (Surowiec et al., 2016).

3. Coronary artery disease is the result of long-term abnormal metabolism called "the metabolic syndrome" (Mottillo et al., 2010 Journ am Coll Cardio).

Blocked communication and miscommunication inhibit the healing cycle, and prevent normal energy, information, and resource-coordination with other organ systems (Wallace, 2010 Proc. Natl. Acad. Sci.). When chronic disease is seen as a systems problem in which the healing system is blocked by malfunction of signaling molecules, new therapeutic approaches become apparent that were hidden before. What follows is a description of our best current model of the metabolic features of the healing cycle.

Change Of States, Phase Change, Equilibrium And Feedback Loops

Your body is complex, you understand that now. The systems of your body work together and affect each other, you understand that now as well. But how does your body maintain itself without any 'central control unit' directed at maintaining all your systems? Once you truly understand that, it will give you a lot of power to support your body's innate ability to heal. Let's dive into some definitions to get to that level of understanding:

- **Irregular Response** refers to the many ways that Allostasis in your body can respond to stress. These changes within your systems are often non-proportionate. i. e. : small changes cause large response and vice versa.

- **Subclinical Change:** This is like when water begins to heat up, but steam has not yet been produced. The water is hotter, but there's no physical evidence yet. Pre-diabetes is like that. It is a subclinical change when your blood sugar rises, but it is before you move into full blown diabetes. Your system wants to remain in a certain physiological range, it wants to hold its 'equilibrium'. Your body uses other systems within itself to keep trying to return to the 'center'. Even though stress keeps disrupting your equilibrium, the body knows how to keep returning. UNTIL . . . it is stressed for too long . . . then it shifts to a new center / equilibrium. When it shifts, that is when imbalance begins.

- **Feedback Loops:** Equilibrium is partly established by the dynamic interchange of both negative and positive feedback. Negative feedback is when a disruption causes change in the *opposite* direction. That is, a thermostat shuts off heat when it's too hot. Positive Feedback is when a disruption causes more change in the *same* direction; i. e., the herd effects. One wolf howls and they all join in. Negative and Positive feedback collaborate. Positive feedback causes a fight or flight response and negative feedback shuts it down when the threat is gone.

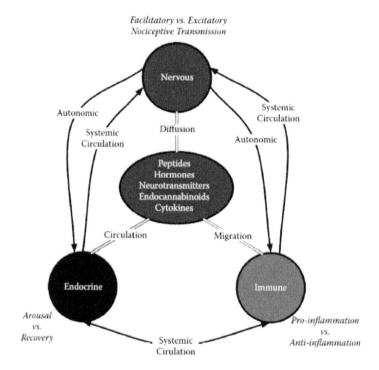

Image from Chapman, et al. Page 37 J Pain.
Author manuscript; PMC 2009 February 1.

SYSTEM COMMUNICATION

This process uses chemicals (center of figure) like hormones, peptides, neurotransmitters, endocannabinoids and cytokines to provide different effects depending on the situation. The communication of all the systems ensures a HOLISTIC response.

The Nervous System detects information from the outside to the spinal cord and brain to process and to provide instructions to the body. It anticipates and detects threats, so we can mobilize our defense.

The Endocrine System hormones in the circulatory system protect the body by fight or flight and encourage healing and recovery when the threat is removed.

The Immune System detects microbial threats in our internal environment and destroys invaders and uses your inflammatory process to heal injuries.

The Circulatory System and Autonomic Nervous System provide information because the nervous, hormone and immune systems need constant, reciprocal communication to respond to stress in an orchestrated manner.

Holistic Systemic Malfunction

When one system malfunctions, its coordination with other systems may also become abnormal.

1. Feedback Loop Dysfunction. Insulin resistance and auto-immune disease are examples of broken negative feedback communication to positive feedback loops.
2. Allostatic Reprioritization. Ongoing stress causes the weakest system link to break down by draining your energy on the stress response. A phenomenon called Pregnenolone steal (aka Cortisol shunt) sets in where cortisol production becomes the predominant pathway of hormone production. Other hormones such as Pregnenolone, DHEA, testosterone and estrogen production suffer a decline.
3. System Shift. A system set point is altered and fails to return to normal causing a new equilibrium to be established. A toxin may cause stress for so long that equilibrium fails to normalize even after stress is removed. Cancer or post - traumatic stress are shifts that cause systemic discoordination.
4. Biorhythm disruption. Biorhythm hormones that control sleep, hunger, rest, sex drive, etc., can get disrupted and malfunction.

System Error or System Correction?

You may have a condition that has traditionally been thought of as a health problem that needs medication- but now through the Systems Approach, common conditions are now being looked at as lifesaving adaptations of your body systems. That is a huge shift in thinking about illness. Your body is responding and trying to heal, yet the current medical system is medicating it to stop the process. Functional Medicine approaches the systems to provide a pathway to allow the lifesaving processes to continue.

1. Euthyroid: classically we approach a sluggish thyroid as illness, but a new model called "Euthyroid Sick Syndrome" is gaining acceptance as a healthy response to a high metabolism that is causing the body to catabolize (eat) itself.
2. Blood pressure: Lowering a reading of 140/90 with drugs increases the risk of dementia in the elderly. The body is trying to pump up circulation to further compartments of the body and brain. Lowering blood pressure to 120 over 80 increases the risk of dementia.
3. Cholesterol: Cholesterol is important to replace damaged cells. In fact, no cell can form without it. So, if you have damaged cells that need to be replaced, your liver is notified to make more cholesterol to release into your blood, so you can make new, healthy cells. If excess damage is occurring, it would not seem very smart to merely lower the cholesterol and forget about why it is high in the first place. It would be wiser to address the cause of the chronic inflammation that is causing damage.

A Note From Dr. Kobsar:

I've wanted to help people with their health as far back as I could remember. I grew up admiring my father's dedication to making a difference as a social worker, presiding over our church council, doing volunteer work and playing hockey until 53 years old. Both of my parents are well into their 80's and continue to work out at the gym three times a week. I became fascinated with wellness while at college and decided I wanted to dedicate my life to helping people by applying the science I learned at university to a natural approach instead of symptom masking medications. I took all my pre-med courses like human anatomy and physiology, skipping the Thursday night parties because I had pop quizzes in chemistry, biology and physics Friday mornings. But I didn't mind! I was excited that I got to learn and grow my brain. I enrolled in a 4-year Doctor of Chiropractic program with the goal to bring my passion for a natural, wellness lifestyle to people who were suffering. But I was still not satisfied. Six months after graduating I was awarded a position that allowed me to apply my research skills and my passion to help people.

I first studied metabolic syndrome in 1996 through a five-year grant I received to work with HIV/AIDS patients in the county hospital system. The patients were very sick, and I witnessed on a daily basis how one of their systems activated and triggered sickness behavior. One system could trigger chronic pain, fatigue, brain fog, digestive stress, insomnia, sexual dysfunction, skin problems and depression. By now, with what you've learned through our book, you can understand how these syndromes are often rooted in the issues discussed in the previous chapters. Many times, an emotional trauma, infection or chemical exposure can be the tipping point that sends your body into imbalance causing a variety of symptoms, but it all is related to your body's inability to produce sufficient energy to do what it is innately designed to do—heal and function optimally!

Case Study: Titan

Titan was sent to us by his doctor with cancer, diabetes, low testosterone, low thyroid and a virus in his eye that required multiple eye surgeries. It seemed like I was going to see him in the Intensive Care Unit every other month. He was on extremely strong medications and we feared that we were going to lose him a few times. When your immune system is taxed by that many diseases, any small problem can blow up and cost you your life. But he hung in there and fought hard. He stuck with our program and in time he turned things around! By adopting our RECREATE Principals, he lowered his allostatic stress by fixing his gut, addressing toxicity, balancing his nutrition, and implementing exercise. He cried in our office, wondering why he had to see five doctors before he could find the answer and regain his health. He got off many of his meds, he got off disability and returned to the work force because we were not simply treating symptoms. We restored his health, so his body could do its job and fight back. He got his family back, his job back, his dignity back and his life back.

Pathways To Premature Aging

Damage shows up as premature aging in your body. Inflammation and an imbalance in your nutrients increase cellular destruction and chronic wasting so regardless of the name of the disease, we know we can help prevent the implications of their destruction.

The drivers of Inflammation are thoroughly discussed in the Inflammation chapter of this book.

The integration between systems is displayed during the response to prolonged activation of the systems from four chronic stressors:

1. Physical trauma
2. Emotional Stress
3. Toxins and Lifestyle Factors
4. The immune system can mistakenly trigger an inflammatory response when no threat is present and chronic low-grade inflammation causing symptoms of allergies, heart disease, cancer, autoimmunity etc. For more, please review the chapter on inflammation.

Nutrients are critical to your health as was thoroughly covered in the Nutrition Chapter of this book.

Preventing Premature Aging

We have yet to meet anyone that wants to age prematurely. In our clinic, our Wellness Partners are committed to gracefully slowing the aging process and living long, vital lives. If you've read this far into our book, then we know you are part of this very exclusive, committed tribe of educated and motivated individuals. Premature aging is driven primarily by your immune-inflammatory response and as you have learned, many factors drive this response. Genetics are out of your control however, you do control more than you think. You control your health choices which create the environment in your body. That environment either stimulates or inhibits your genetic expression of risk factors. You have learned that if you have system dysregulation causing a chronic disease such as anxiety, irritable bowel syndrome, multiple sclerosis or diabetes, the conditions will not be resolved by a single symptom solution like medication. The problem must be addressed at a global level i. e. : hormones, diet, sleep, exercise, toxic burden, or stress reduction. From a systems perspective, we look at disease as involving a phase change in the health of the system brought on by ongoing stressors with enough time to wear down the adaptive capacities. We must break a stuck feedback loop to restore balance or we will continue to suffer from chronic disease. However, if you systematically balance each of your systems with what you have learned in this book, you will eventually reset your entire life.

SYSTEMIC DYSREGULATION AND METABOLIC DEGENERATION

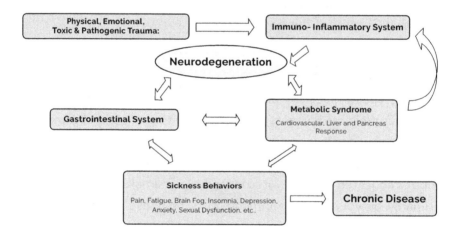

HOLISTIC MEDICINE

This entire chapter has been a discussion of the very essence of Holistic Medicine where the whole body is considered rather than broken into separate parts or pieces. Systems coordinate a defense response that can be set to higher or lower levels of tolerance. For the sensitive person, any amount of stress causes a strong response. The person feels sickness with only minor stress because they have endured years of chronic stress. Other people have a defense system that can tolerate massive stress. They run marathons or work 60 hours a week with no dip in energy, vitality and well-being. It all comes down to how much energy is drained on a daily basis. Ongoing stress can cause a phase shift in our defense systems, making us hyperactive but systems shift back to a healthier set point through lifestyle improvements over time. Progress may be hard to measure because complex systems often change in a 'two steps forward, one step back' fashion making it difficult to assess. The answer is not to focus on one isolated event but instead, look at overall trends and the trajectory of your health. If you slowly push that change long enough, you can get over the hump (system shift) and cause a big jump in progress and establish a new set point.

Conventional healthcare treats each component of each syndrome separately, with emphasis on the parts that respond to medication. The trouble with this approach is that there are typically a number of causes of disease. We can't just ignore the underlying cause and settle for treating symptoms. We are not saying to let people suffer and not treat symptoms, we are not saying that you just don't stop searching for the cause. We speak with too many patients who were told their disease was due to their age, genetics, or labelled with some "syndrome", and with no solutions- so they settled on symptom care with medications.

Metabolic addiction to the chemistry produced by the Cell Danger Response can occur which can create a life-long risk of relapse if diet and lifestyle interventions are not maintained. Prevention and treatment of chronic illness require distinctly different approaches. New cases of chronic illness can be *prevented* by reducing the environmental risks that trigger the damage cycle of the CDR, and by promoting life-style changes that promote resilience and maintain health. However, once illness occurs, the opportunity for prevention is lost, and a perfect storm of triggers can usually be identified. Many triggers are remote and no longer present. Once any remaining triggers have been identified and removed, and any symptoms or primed sensitivities caused by the metabolic memory of those triggers have been treated, a new approach to *treatment* is required to improve the chances of completing the healing cycle and achieving a full recovery. By shifting the focus to the metabolic factors and signaling pathways that *maintain* chronic illness by blocking progress through the healing cycle, new treatments will follow.

Despite the complaints from patients to their doctors, routine blood tests are surprisingly normal, an indicator their syndromes are outside the available testing in many clinics. It is important not to give up and accept that 'everything' has been done. There are life-changing tests that identify abnormalities at the root of diminishing metabolic function not being used in conventional medicine. The ion exchange test for brain function provides clues that standard blood labs do not. Functional Medicine has established parameters of blood lab interpretations based on optimal health of the body. With the introduction of inexpensive methods for measuring telomeres, we can now integrate genetic data and study how metabolic degeneration, normal aging, system dysregulation all interact to affect gene expression.

CONCLUSION

Treating systems can be overwhelming at first so don't try to treat everything at once. But, we can succeed by using a comprehensive approach to inhibit allostatic stress overload and metabolic degeneration by emphasizing building blocks for an anabolic metabolism. **Detoxification** is an anabolic process where our body produces enzymes to address toxins. Chronically ill patients lose their ability to detoxify their body. The body reprioritizes resources when inflammation is high, and we see a drop of phase 1 and phase 2 detoxification enzymes, loss of methylation and catecholamine methyltransferase ability needed for estrogen metabolism. Inflammation and stress redirect your body's resources away from non-life-threatening conditions like osteoporosis, blood sugar, sex hormone production, etc. . . . to more critical concerns like brain, heart and liver disease. A lifetime of stress has cumulative effects on your allostatic systems.

Inflammatory stressors and energy conservation are a great place to start. There is not one most important stressor. All are equally important, depending on the severity of the stressor. They all create inflammation. Food is energy and our metabolic use of energy can create order out of chaos. Introducing a systems approach to allostatic overload sets people up for long term success and better treatment outcomes. We don't expect you to be completely free from stress. You can't live in a bubble free from toxins, eat plants every day and exercise 7 times a week forever. Life happens, we know this. But you can balance your systems and lower your allostatic stress by working each one of the RECREATE Principles into your life slowly, over time. If you have come this far it is likely you have already taken some steps forward and we want to encourage you to keep the momentum going forward and take some more steps.

We hope you enjoyed this deep dive and are ready to apply all that you learned to your health and your life. However, we want to strongly encourage you not to make the mistake of waiting to start taking action. Too many people get caught up in the 'paralysis of analysis' and confuse learning more with actually doing something about their

health. You have been given knowledge, wisdom and action steps to RECREATE your health. Remember that knowledge is only power when you act on it, otherwise it is worthless-
so get going—its time!

To your good health!
Dr. Bradley Kobsar and Judy Pearson Kobsar

Made in the USA
Las Vegas, NV
01 April 2021